Elder Abuse and Its Prevention

Workshop Summary

Rachel M. Taylor, *Rapporteur*

Forum on Global Violence Prevention

Board on Global Health

INSTITUTE OF MEDICINE AND
NATIONAL RESEARCH COUNCIL
OF THE NATIONAL ACADEMIES

THE NATIONAL ACADEMIES PRESS
Washington, D.C.
www.nap.edu

THE NATIONAL ACADEMIES PRESS   500 Fifth Street, NW   Washington, DC 20001

NOTICE: The workshop that is the subject of this workshop summary was approved by the Governing Board of the National Research Council, whose members are drawn from the councils of the National Academy of Sciences, the National Academy of Engineering, and the Institute of Medicine.

This workshop summary was supported by contracts between the National Academy of Sciences and the Department of Health and Human Services: Administration on Aging, Office on Women's Health; Anheuser-Busch InBev; the Archstone Foundation; the Avon Foundation for Women; BD (Becton, Dickinson and Company); Catholic Health Initiatives; the Centers for Disease Control and Prevention; the Department of Justice: National Institute of Justice; Eli Lilly and Company; the F Felix Foundation; the Fetzer Institute; the Foundation to Promote Open Society; the Joyce Foundation; John E. Fogarty International Center; Kaiser Permanente; LeadingAge; Merck & Co., Inc.; the National Institutes of Health: National Institute on Alcoholism and Alcohol Abuse, National Institute on Drug Abuse, Office of Research on Women's Health; the Robert Wood Johnson Foundation; and Wells Fargo Advisors. The views presented in this summary do not necessarily reflect the views of the organizations or agencies that provided support for the activity.

International Standard Book Number-13: 978-0-309-29351-8
International Standard Book Number-10: 0-309-29351-0

Additional copies of this workshop summary are available from the National Academies Press, 500 Fifth Street, NW, Keck 360, Washington, DC 20001; (800) 624-6242 or (202) 334-3313; http://www.nap.edu.

For more information about the Institute of Medicine, visit the IOM home page at: www.iom.edu.

Copyright 2014 by the National Academy of Sciences. All rights reserved.

Printed in the United States of America

The serpent has been a symbol of long life, healing, and knowledge among almost all cultures and religions since the beginning of recorded history. The serpent adopted as a logotype by the Institute of Medicine is a relief carving from ancient Greece, now held by the Staatliche Museen in Berlin.

Suggested citation: IOM (Institute of Medicine) and NRC (National Research Council). 2014. *Elder abuse and its prevention: Workshop summary.* Washington, DC: The National Academies Press.

THE NATIONAL ACADEMIES
Advisers to the Nation on Science, Engineering, and Medicine

The **National Academy of Sciences** is a private, nonprofit, self-perpetuating society of distinguished scholars engaged in scientific and engineering research, dedicated to the furtherance of science and technology and to their use for the general welfare. Upon the authority of the charter granted to it by the Congress in 1863, the Academy has a mandate that requires it to advise the federal government on scientific and technical matters. Dr. Ralph J. Cicerone is president of the National Academy of Sciences.

The **National Academy of Engineering** was established in 1964, under the charter of the National Academy of Sciences, as a parallel organization of outstanding engineers. It is autonomous in its administration and in the selection of its members, sharing with the National Academy of Sciences the responsibility for advising the federal government. The National Academy of Engineering also sponsors engineering programs aimed at meeting national needs, encourages education and research, and recognizes the superior achievements of engineers. Dr. C. D. Mote, Jr., is president of the National Academy of Engineering.

The **Institute of Medicine** was established in 1970 by the National Academy of Sciences to secure the services of eminent members of appropriate professions in the examination of policy matters pertaining to the health of the public. The Institute acts under the responsibility given to the National Academy of Sciences by its congressional charter to be an adviser to the federal government and, upon its own initiative, to identify issues of medical care, research, and education. Dr. Harvey V. Fineberg is president of the Institute of Medicine.

The **National Research Council** was organized by the National Academy of Sciences in 1916 to associate the broad community of science and technology with the Academy's purposes of furthering knowledge and advising the federal government. Functioning in accordance with general policies determined by the Academy, the Council has become the principal operating agency of both the National Academy of Sciences and the National Academy of Engineering in providing services to the government, the public, and the scientific and engineering communities. The Council is administered jointly by both Academies and the Institute of Medicine. Dr. Ralph J. Cicerone and Dr. C. D. Mote, Jr., are chair and vice chair, respectively, of the National Research Council.

www.national-academies.org

PLANNING COMMITTEE FOR WORKSHOP ON ELDER ABUSE AND ITS PREVENTION[1]

JACQUELYN C. CAMPBELL (*Co-Chair*), Anna D. Wolf Chair and Professor, Johns Hopkins University School of Nursing
XINQI DONG (*Co-Chair*), Associate Director, Rush Institute for Health Aging; Associate Professor of Medicine, Behavioral Sciences, and Gerontological Nursing, Rush University Medical Center
TERRY T. FULMER, Dean, Bouvé College of Health Sciences, Northeastern University
JEFFREY E. HALL, Behavioral Scientist and Acting Team Lead, Morbidity and Behavioral Surveillance Team Surveillance Branch, Division of Violence Prevention, National Center for Injury Prevention and Control, Centers for Disease Control and Prevention
ALEXANDRE KALACHE, President, International Longevity Centre–Brazil
TARA L. McMULLEN, Health Analyst, Quality Measures & Health Assessment Group, Center for Clinical Standards and Quality, Centers for Medicare & Medicaid Services
EDWIN L. WALKER, Deputy Assistant Secretary, Program Operations, Administration on Aging

---

[1] Institute of Medicine planning committees are solely responsible for organizing the workshop, identifying topics, and choosing speakers. The responsibility for the published workshop summary rests with the workshop rapporteur and the institution.

FORUM ON GLOBAL VIOLENCE PREVENTION[1]

JACQUELYN C. CAMPBELL (*Co-Chair*), Anna D. Wolf Chair and Professor, Johns Hopkins University School of Nursing
MARK L. ROSENBERG (*Co-Chair*), President and Chief Executive Officer, The Task Force for Global Health
ALBERT J. ALLEN, Senior Medical Fellow, Bioethics and Pediatric Capabilities, Global Medical Affairs and Development Center of Excellence, Eli Lilly and Company
CLARE ANDERSON, Deputy Commissioner, Administration on Children, Youth and Families, Department of Health and Human Services (until June 2013)
FRANCES ASHE-GOINS, Deputy Director, Office on Women's Health, Department of Health and Human Services
KATRINA BAUM, Senior Research Officer, Office of Research Partnerships, National Institute of Justice, Department of Justice (until January 2014)
SUSAN BISSELL, Associate Director, Child Protection Section, United Nations Children's Fund
ARTURO CERVANTES TREJO, Professor and Chair of Public Health, Anahuac Institute of Public Health, Mexico
XINQI DONG, Associate Director, Rush Institute for Health Aging; Associate Professor of Medicine, Behavioral Sciences, and Gerontological Nursing, Rush University Medical Center
AMIE GIANINO, Senior Global Director, Beer & Better World, Anheuser-Busch InBev (until December 2013)
KATHY GREENLEE, Assistant Secretary for Aging, Administration on Aging, Department of Health and Human Services
GENE GUERRERO, Director, Crime and Violence Prevention Initiative, Open Society Foundations (until June 2013)
RODRIGO V. GUERRERO, Mayor, Cali, Colombia
DAVID HEMENWAY, Professor of Health Policy; Director, Injury Control Research Center and the Youth Violence Prevention Center, Harvard University School of Public Health
FRANCES HENRY, Advisor, F Felix Foundation
LARKE NAHME HUANG, Senior Advisor, Office of the Administrator, Substance Abuse and Mental Health Services Administration, Department of Health and Human Services (until June 2013)

---

[1] Institute of Medicine forums and roundtables do not issue, review, or approve individual documents. The responsibility for the published workshop summary rests with the workshop rapporteur and the institution.

L. ROWELL HUESMANN, Amos N. Tversky Collegiate Professor of Psychology and Communication Studies; Director, Research Center for Group Dynamics, Institute for Social Research, University of Michigan
CAROL M. KURZIG, President, Avon Foundation for Women
JACQUELINE LLOYD, Health Scientist Administrator, National Institute on Drug Abuse, National Institutes of Health, Department of Health and Human Services (until June 2013)
JANE ISAACS LOWE, Senior Advisor for Program Development, Robert Wood Johnson Foundation
BRIGID McCAW, Medical Director, NCal Family Violence Prevention Program, Kaiser Permanente
JAMES A. MERCY, Special Advisor for Strategic Directions, Division of Violence Prevention, National Center for Injury Prevention and Control, Centers for Disease Control and Prevention
MICHELE MOLONEY-KITTS, Managing Director, Together for Girls
LAURA MOSQUEDA, Associate Dean of Primary Care, University of California, Irvine, School of Medicine
MARGARET M. MURRAY, Director, Global Alcohol Research Program, National Institute on Alcohol Abuse and Alcoholism, National Institutes of Health, Department of Health and Human Services
MICHAEL PHILLIPS, Director, Suicide Research and Prevention Center, Shanghai Jiao Tong University School of Medicine
COLLEEN SCANLON, Senior Vice President, Advocacy, Catholic Health Initiatives
EVELYN TOMASZEWSKI, Senior Policy Advisor, Human Rights and International Affairs, National Association of Social Workers
ELIZABETH WARD, Chair, Violence Prevention Alliance, University of the West Indies, Mona Campus

IOM Staff

RACHEL M. TAYLOR, Associate Program Officer
MEGAN M. PEREZ, Research Assistant
AUDREY AVILA, Intern
NIKITA SRINIVASAN, Intern
CHRISTEN WOODS, Intern
DEEPALI M. PATEL, Program Officer (until February 2013)
KIMBERLY SCOTT, Senior Program Officer (from June 2013)
KATHERINE M. BLAKESLEE, IPA
MELISSA A. SIMON, Institute of Medicine Anniversary Fellow
JULIE WILTSHIRE, Financial Officer
PATRICK W. KELLEY, Senior Board Director, Board on Global Health

Reviewers

This workshop summary has been reviewed in draft form by individuals chosen for their diverse perspectives and technical expertise, in accordance with procedures approved by the National Research Council's Report Review Committee. The purpose of this independent review is to provide candid and critical comments that will assist the institution in making its published report as sound as possible and to ensure that the workshop summary meets institutional standards for objectivity, evidence, and responsiveness to the study charge. The review comments and draft manuscript remain confidential to protect the integrity of the process. We wish to thank the following individuals for their review of this report:

GEORGIA J. ANETZBERGER, Cleveland State University
CLAUDIA COOPER, University College London
JEFFREY HALL, Centers for Disease Control and Prevention
PAMELA TEASTER, University of Kentucky

Although the reviewers listed above have provided many constructive comments and suggestions, they did not see the final draft of the workshop summary before its release. The review of this workshop summary was overseen by **David B. Reuben,** University of California, Los Angeles. Appointed by the Institute of Medicine, he was responsible for making certain that an independent examination of this workshop summary was carried out in accordance with institutional procedures and that all review comments were carefully considered. Responsibility for the final content of this workshop summary rests entirely with the rapporteur and the institution.

Acknowledgments

The Forum on Global Violence Prevention was established to develop multisectoral collaboration among stakeholders. Violence prevention is a cross-disciplinary field that could benefit from increased dialogue among researchers, policy makers, funders, and practitioners. As awareness of the insidious and pervasive nature of violence grows, so too does the imperative to mitigate and prevent it. The Forum seeks to illuminate and explore evidence-based approaches to the prevention of violence.

A number of individuals contributed to the development of this workshop and report. These include a number of staff members from the Institute of Medicine and the National Academies: Charlee Alexander, Daniel Bethea, Karen Campion, Leigh Carroll, Marton Cavani, Colin Fink, Meg Ginivan, Wendy Keenan, Patrick Kelley, Jillian Laffrey, Eileen Milner, Crysti Park, Jose Portillo, Patsy Powell, and Julie Wiltshire. The Forum staff, including Megan Perez, Kimberly Scott, and Rachel Taylor, put forth considerable effort to ensure this workshop's success.

The planning committee contributed hours of service to develop and execute the agenda, with the guidance of Forum membership. Reviewers also provided thoughtful remarks in reading the draft manuscript. Finally, these efforts would not be possible without the work of the Forum membership itself, an esteemed body of individuals dedicated to the concept that violence is preventable.

This workshop was made possible through the support of the Forum sponsors and the workshop sponsors: Cedar Village, Cincinnati; The Hebrew Home at Riverdale; the Jewish Home of Fairfield County, Connecticut; LeadingAge; Merck & Co., Inc.; and Wells Fargo Advisors.

The overall successful functioning of the Forum and its activities depends on the generosity of its sponsors. Financial support for the Forum on Global Violence Prevention is provided by the Department of Health and Human Services: Administration on Aging, Office on Women's Health; Anheuser-Busch InBev; the Archstone Foundation; the Avon Foundation for Women; BD (Becton, Dickinson and Company); Catholic Health Initiatives; the Centers for Disease Control and Prevention; the Department of Justice: National Institute of Justice; Eli Lilly and Company; the F Felix Foundation; the Fetzer Institute; the Foundation to Promote Open Society; the Joyce Foundation; John E. Fogarty International Center; Kaiser Permanente; the National Institutes of Health: National Institute on Alcoholism and Alcohol Abuse, National Institute on Drug Abuse, Office of Research on Women's Health; and the Robert Wood Johnson Foundation.

Contents

PART I: WORKSHOP OVERVIEW

1	Introduction	1
2	Measuring and Conceptualizing Elder Abuse	6
3	Risk Factors and Health Outcomes	18
4	Ethical Considerations	25
5	Screening and Prevention	31
6	The Way Forward	41

PART II: PAPERS AND COMMENTARY FROM SPEAKERS

II.1	Understanding Elder Abuse in the Chinese Community: The Role of Cultural, Social, and Community Factors *E-Shien* **Chang** *and XinQi* **Dong**	53
II.2	Seven Policy Priorities for an Enhanced Public Health Response to Elder Abuse *Marie-Therese* **Connolly** *and Ariel Trilling*	59
II.3	Elder Neglect: The State of the Science *Terry T.* **Fulmer** *and XinQi* **Dong**	67
II.4	Native Elder Mistreatment *Lori L.* **Jervis**	75
II.5	Elder Financial Abuse *Ronald* **Long**	80

II.6	Elder Abuse and Its Prevention: Screening and Detection *Tara **McMullen**, Kimberly **Schwartz**, Mark **Yaffe**, and Scott **Beach***	88
II.7	Elder Abuse and Neglect: A Role for Physicians *James G. **O'Brien***	94
II.8	Preventing Elder Abuse—Hope Springs Eternal *Elizabeth **Podnieks** and Cynthia Thomas*	95
II.9	Elder Abuse Intervention: The Shelter Model and the Long-Term Care Facility *Daniel A. **Reingold**, Joy **Solomon**, and Malya Levin*	101
II.10	Elder Abuse in Asia—An Overview *Elsie **Yan***	105

APPENDIXES

A	Workshop Agenda	125
B	Speaker Biographical Sketches	133

Part I

Workshop Overview

1

Introduction[1]

Elder abuse is a violation on older adults' fundamental rights to be safe and free from violence and contradicts efforts toward improved well-being and quality of life in healthy aging. Data suggest that 1 in 10 older adults in the United States experience physical, psychological, or sexual abuse, neglect, or financial exploitation. In low- and middle-income countries, where the burden of violence is the greatest, prevalence is likely higher. Predictions indicate that by 2050, 22 percent of the world population will be 60 years or older, doubling the 2009 global population of older adults (UN, 2009). However, despite the magnitude of elder abuse globally, it has been an underappreciated public health problem. Resources allocated toward understanding elder abuse and effective interventions for preventing it are often limited and fall short of those applied to more recognized public health problems.

On April 17 and 18, 2013, the Institute of Medicine's (IOM's) Forum on Global Violence Prevention convened a 2-day workshop on elder abuse and its prevention (see Box 1-1 for the Statement of Task). Part of the Forum's mandate is to engage in multisectoral, multidirectional dialogue that explores crosscutting approaches to violence prevention. While elder

---

[1] The planning committee's role was limited to planning the workshop. The workshop summary was prepared by the rapporteur as a factual summary of what occurred at the workshop. Statements, recommendations, and opinions expressed are those of individual presenters and participants and are not necessarily endorsed or verified by the Forum on Global Violence Prevention, the Institute of Medicine, or the National Research Council, and they should not be construed as reflecting any group consensus.

> **BOX 1-1**
> **Statement of Task**
> **Elder Abuse and Its Prevention: A Workshop**
>
> Violence and related forms of abuse against elders is a global public health and human rights problem with far-reaching consequences, resulting in increased death, disability, and exploitation with collateral effects on well-being. Data suggest that at least 10 percent of elders in the United States are victims of elder maltreatment every year. In low- and middle-income countries, where the burden of violence is the greatest, the figure is likely even higher. In addition, elders experiencing risk factors such as diminishing cognitive function, caregiver dependence, and social isolation are more vulnerable to maltreatment and underreporting. As the world population of adults aged 65 and older continues to grow, the implications of elder maltreatment for health care, social welfare, justice, and financial systems are great. However, despite the magnitude of global elder maltreatment, it has been an underappreciated public health problem.
>
> The Institute of Medicine will host a 2-day public workshop on global elder abuse and its prevention. Using an ecological framework, this workshop will explore the burden of elder abuse around the world, focusing on its impacts on individuals, families, communities, and societies. Additionally, the workshop will address occurrences and co-occurrences of different types of abuse, including physical, sexual, emotional, and financial, as well as neglect. The ultimate objective is to illuminate promising global and multisectoral evidence-based approaches to the prevention of elder maltreatment.
>
> The workshop will be planned and conducted by an ad hoc committee that will develop the workshop agenda, select and invite speakers and discussants, and moderate the discussions. Experts will be drawn from the public and private sectors as well as from academic organizations to allow for multilateral, evidence-based discussions. Following the conclusion of the workshop, an individually authored summary of the event will be prepared by a designated rapporteur. The workshop will be free and open to the public.

abuse has been addressed in previous Forum workshops,[2] it has lacked the attention that some other forms of violence, such as child abuse and sexual violence, have received. The Forum chose to dedicate a workshop to elder abuse and its prevention to shed light on this underappreciated and often overlooked form of violence. This workshop was an opportunity to engage

---

[2] Previous Forum on Global Violence Prevention workshop summaries include *Preventing Violence Against Women and Children* (IOM and NRC, 2011); *Social and Economic Costs of Violence* (IOM and NRC, 2012a); *Communications and Technology for Violence Prevention* (IOM and NRC, 2012b); *Contagion of Violence* (IOM and NRC, 2013); and *Evidence for Violence Prevention Across the Lifespan and Around the World* (IOM and NRC, 2014). All Forum workshop summaries and additional information on previous workshops are available at http://www.iom.edu/globalviolenceprevention.

in a more comprehensive discussion of the global burden of elder abuse and how to prevent it. Considering the limited awareness of the magnitude of elder abuse, even within the violence prevention community, workshop speakers discussed the prevalence and characteristics of elder abuse around the world, risk factors for abuse and potential adverse health outcomes, and contextually specific factors, such as culture and the role of the community.

Elder abuse has several aspects that are unique from other forms of violence. These unique aspects deserve specific illumination, such as the role of cognitive impairment and social isolation. Thus, workshop speakers highlighted these aspects in terms of ethical considerations in research and practice and rights versus protection of older adults. While the workshop covered scope and prevalence and unique characteristics of abuse, the intention was to move beyond what is known about elder abuse to foster discussions about how to improve prevention, intervention, and mitigation of the victims' needs, particularly through collaborative efforts. Therefore the workshop discussions included innovative intervention models and opportunities for prevention across sectors and settings. These discussions are covered in this summary report.

DEFINITIONS AND CONTEXT

Within the field of elder abuse, different terms are used to define the parameters of violence, abuse, neglect, self-neglect, and exploitation of the elderly as described within specific context. For example, the 2003 National Research Council report *Elder Mistreatment: Abuse, Neglect, and Exploitation in an Aging America* defined elder mistreatment "as (a) intentional actions that cause harm or create serious risk of harm (whether or not harm is intended) to a vulnerable elder by a caregiver or other person who stands in a trust relationship to the elder or (b) failure by a caregiver to satisfy the elder's basic needs or to protect the elder from harm" (NRC, 2003, p. 1). For specificity of context, this definition is intended to exclude cases of self-neglect and cases involving victimization of elders by strangers (p. 1). The World Health Organization uses the term "elder abuse" and has adopted the definition developed in 1995 by Action on Elder Abuse in the United Kingdom: "elder abuse is a single or repeated act or lack of appropriate action, occurring within any relationship where there is an expectation of trust which causes harm or distress to an older person" (WHO, 2008, p. 6). Still others use the term "elder maltreatment," borrowing from the field of child maltreatment in which maltreatment "refers to the physical and emotional mistreatment, sexual abuse, neglect and negligent treatment of children, as well as to their commercial or other exploitation" (WHO and International Society for Prevention of Child Abuse and Neglect, 2006). However, there are no standard, universally accepted definitions of elder abuse, elder mistreatment, or elder maltreatment. While this report highlights some of the issues with a lack of common definitions, as well as ongoing efforts to establish them, it does not attempt to resolve them. Rather, as a summary report, terminology is applied based on the language used by the individual speakers and participants. In text that is not directly attributable to individual speakers and participants, the term elder abuse is applied.

ORGANIZATION OF THE REPORT

This report provides a summary account of the presentations given at the workshop and expert papers submitted by workshop speakers. Opinions expressed within this summary are not those of the IOM, the Forum on Global Violence Prevention, or their agents, but rather of the presenters themselves. Such statements are the views of the speakers and do not reflect conclusions or recommendations of a formally appointed committee. This summary was authored by a designated rapporteur based on the workshop presentations and discussions and does not represent the views of the institution, nor does it constitute a full or exhaustive overview of the field.

The workshop summary is organized thematically, covering the major topics that arose during the 2-day workshop, to present these issues in a larger context and in a compelling and comprehensive way. The thematic organization also allows the summary to serve as an overview of important issues in the field; however, such an organization results in some repetition, as themes are interrelated and the presented examples support several different themes and subthemes raised by speakers. The themes presented in this summary were the frequent and crosscutting elements that arose from the various workshop presentations, but the choice of these themes does not represent any formal consensus process.

The first part of this report consists of an introduction and five chapters, which provide a summary of the workshop; the second part consists of submitted papers from speakers on the substance of the work they presented. These papers were solicited from speakers in order to offer further information about their work and illuminate how such contributions can advance the field of elder abuse prevention; not all speakers contributed papers. The appendixes contain additional information regarding the agenda and participants.

REFERENCES

IOM (Institute of Medicine) and NRC (National Research Council). 2011. *Preventing violence against women and children: Workshop summary.* Washington, DC: The National Academies Press.

IOM and NRC. 2012a. *Social and economic costs of violence: Workshop summary.* Washington, DC: The National Academies Press.
IOM and NRC. 2012b. *Communications and technology for violence prevention: Workshop summary.* Washington, DC: The National Academies Press.
IOM and NRC. 2013. *Contagion of violence: Workshop summary.* Washington, DC: The National Academies Press.
IOM and NRC. 2014. *Evidence for violence prevention across the lifespan and around the world: Workshop summary.* Washington, DC: The National Academies Press.
NRC. 2003. *Elder mistreatment: Abuse, neglect, and exploitation in an aging America.* Washington, DC: The National Academies Press.
UN (United Nations). 2009. *World population ageing.* Department of Economic and Social Affairs, Population Division. New York: UN.
WHO (World Health Organization). 2008. *A global response to elder abuse and neglect: Building primary health care capacity to deal with the problem worldwide: Main report.* Geneva, Switzerland: WHO.
WHO and International Society for Prevention of Child Abuse and Neglect. 2006. *Preventing child maltreatment: A guide to taking action and generating evidence.* Geneva, Switzerland: WHO.

2

Measuring and Conceptualizing Elder Abuse

Measuring elder abuse is challenging, as definitions and conceptualizations of what constitutes elder abuse vary across disciplines, sectors, and cultures. The lack of common definitions and conceptualization of elder abuse and the need for common ground to better understand and collect data on elder abuse were raised by several workshop speakers. As workshop speaker Robert Wallace from the University of Iowa commented, "The problem is, if we do not count cases with good definitions, we cannot know how many people there are. If we do not know that, we do not know whether the [intervention] program works."

Speaker and planning committee member Tara McMullen from the Centers for Medicare & Medicaid Services noted that even across U.S. government agencies, definitions of elder abuse and how it is classified vary. As acknowledged by the Centers for Disease Control and Prevention, "elder abuse has been (1) poorly or imprecisely defined, (2) defined specifically to reflect the unique statutes or conditions present in specific locations (e.g., states, counties, or cities), or (3) defined specifically for research purposes. As a result, a set of universally accepted definitions does not exist" (CDC, 2013).

Although how elder abuse was defined varied, the categories of abuse discussed at the workshop included physical, sexual, emotional, and financial, as well as neglect and self-neglect. Several speakers also raised some culturally specific types of abuse, such as exclusion from participation in cultural activities. In addition to varying definitions and concepts, measuring and ultimately preventing elder abuse is complicated by several other factors that were raised by workshop speakers: the setting and cultural context in which it occurs; the role of cognitive impairment; unique challenges in terms of neglect and self-neglect; and lack of a common conceptual framework.

SETTINGS

Several speakers noted that there are not only differences in types of abuse, but that it occurs in different settings, primarily differentiating between community and institutional settings. Workshop speakers presented findings from research on elder abuse in both the community and institutions and the implications for each.

Abuse Occurring in the Community

Workshop speaker Ron Acierno from the University of South Carolina presented findings from the National Elder Mistreatment Study, which surveyed community-presiding older adults in the United States. The study found that the rate of elder mistreatment in the community was 10 to 11 percent, not including financial exploitation. Acierno noted that the majority of the violence in the community is domestic violence. He further noted that the participants in this study gave consent to participate, and therefore the rates of dementia among the participants were limited, if at all present. He suggested that because little is known about the effects or remedies for elder abuse within the community, this high rate of mistreatment among community-residing, primarily non-demented, older adults was very concerning.

Several workshop speakers commented on the complexities of elder abuse in the community. The role of family members who may be caregivers and/or abusers, issues of neglect and self-neglect, cultural perceptions of elder abuse within the family, and stigma were all raised as contributors to elder abuse in the community.

Domestic violence in which victims are community-residing older adults has a unique set of challenges from other forms of domestic violence. Administration on Aging Assistant Secretary Kathy Greenlee, a workshop speaker and Forum member, commented that often older adults who are being abused need other services. She asked the audience, "How do you [plan care] for them? Or [do] safety planning? How do you continue to support someone who is a victim of domestic [violence] and is 75 or 85?" These issues need to be addressed in the context of community-residing victims of elder abuse.

Cultural Context

Workshop planning committee co-chair and Forum member XinQi Dong, from the Rush Institute for Healthy Aging, noted that elder abuse in the community setting is further complicated by the sociocultural context. Within the areas of elder abuse research, practice, and policy, he suggested that consideration of culture issues needs to be included to effectively address the needs of the individuals within their communities. Workshop speaker Lori L. Jervis of the University of Oklahoma commented on cultural relativity and the importance of not making assumptions about how types of abuse are perceived within different cultures. For example, she noted that one type of abuse within Native American populations is spiritual abuse. Being denied access to ceremonies that the group finds essential or important and being denied access to a traditional healer when one is sick are examples of what Native American people consider abusive that other populations may not. From her research within the Native American populations, Jervis found that elders see good treatment as a mixture of being taking care of, having one's needs met, and being respected. (For more information on Native American populations and elder abuse, see *Jervis* in Part II of this report.)

Workshop speaker Elsie Yan from the University of Hong Kong noted that, in Chinese populations, disrespect and being ignored or left out of family gatherings are major forms of elder abuse. In Chinese American populations, psychological abuse is considered worse than physical abuse; disrespect, cursing, and ignoring are seen as worse than hitting or other types of physical abuse. In Korean and Indian populations, older adults tend to have high tolerance for financial abuse, as it is common practice for older people to transfer their property and valuables to their adult children in hopes that they would take care of them as they age. In many cases, that does not happen. (For more information on elder abuse in Asia, see *Yan* in Part II of this report.)

Consistent with findings presented by other workshop speakers, Jervis noted that within the Native American populations, she has observed that elder abuse occurs most frequently within a family. Workshop speaker Charles Mouton from Meharry Medical College commented on the complexity of family and community relationships in the reporting of elder abuse. In the context of African American families, older adults often want their children nearby, even if they are being abused by them. They often are reluctant to report abuse because they do not want to harm their family's reputation in the community, or be seen as going against their kin. Jervis and speaker E-Shien Chang from the Rush Institute for Healthy Aging also commented on this issue of family stigma as a barrier to reporting in Native American and Chinese communities, respectively. Often, there is a perception that what happens in the family should stay in the family, and reporting abuse could embarrass the family in front of the larger community.

Chang noted that there is a unique aspect of the perception of elder abuse within Chinese communities that stems from the Confucian belief in filial piety, which dictates children's obligatory roles and responsibilities of caregiving to aging parents. Traditionally, filial piety is expected of adult children and there is a high expectation of emotional support. However, modernization has led to more mobility of adult children from rural to urban settings, affecting traditional family structures and intergenerational caregiving. Within Chinese American communities, filial piety is being affected by a shift from the traditional Chinese conception of collectivism towards the Western individualistic tradition. The discrepancy of expectation versus the receipt of the filial piety made predispose older Chinese Americans to consequences of elder abuse. (For more information on elder abuse and Chinese communities, see *Chang and Dong* in Part II of this report.)

Social Support and the Community

In the context of culture, community and social support play a large role in an older adult's well-being. Throughout the workshop, low social support, or a lack of social connectedness and connectedness to the community, was mentioned as a risk factor for elder abuse. Acierno and colleagues (2010) found low social support as a risk factor for emotional, physical, and sexual mistreatment, as well as neglect. Mouton noted that, within African American communities, abuse is greater among those who are socially isolated; a lack of familiar social networks puts them at somewhat higher risk for abuse.

The issue of migration combined with social isolation and low social support was discussed by several participants. Yan noted that aging migrants often live in communities without family members in close proximity. Forum member Michael Phillips from Shanghai Jiao Tong University School of Medicine commented that, in mainland China, young people are migrating away from the rural areas and into cities, leaving their aging parents behind. Workshop planning committee member Alexander Kalache from the International Longevity Centre–Brazil suggested that the issue of migration is complex; some individuals migrate because they are in search of work and entrepreneurial opportunities, while others migrate because they are persecuted in their home country. These are quite different experiences and the impacts on social support vary. In situations where a community migrates together, they tend to stay together, have extremely close links, and often look out for each other. He suggested that, in terms of the issue of migration and social support, the location of one's birth is not what matters, but rather the density of individuals from the same cultural background who are in one's community.

Yan mentioned additional factors that are affecting social isolation of older adults: environmental and structural changes to communities. In China, the government is removing older community dwellings and developing new buildings. Through the relocation process, older adults who used to have a very good social network in their communities and buildings are losing their social supports.

Abuse Occurring in Institutions

Workshop speaker Mark Lachs from Weill Medical College of Cornell University presented on elder abuse occurring in nursing home facilities. Although reports of elders being abused by nursing home staff have been sensationalized in the media and used to sway public opinion, close some facilities, and require background checks, Lachs suggested that major forms of violence in long-term care that pose the greatest threat to residents go unaddressed.

In the 1970s in New York state, there were descriptions of abuse committed by staff and legislation was passed to protect nursing home residents. About 15 or 20 years ago, a small amount of literature began to emerge about residents themselves committing violence against staff. In this research, staff were asked if they had been physically assaulted by their residents. About 50 percent of the staff described being physically assaulted in the course of providing care to residents. There is also literature about rates of staff-to-staff aggression. More recently, research has been being conducted on resident-to-resident aggression. Figure 2-1 is a model Lachs presented to show the types of violence occurring in nursing homes and the actual level of harm (as opposed to the perceived level) to residents.

Lachs commented on staff-to-resident and resident-to-resident violence from his experience. "I have spent tens of thousands of hours in nursing homes as a physician," he said. "I have never physically seen a staff member strike a resident with my own eyes. Yet every day, I see residents saying bad things or physically striking one another." In addition, Lachs suggested that resident-to-staff abuse may put residents at risk if poorly trained staff retaliate.

Lachs presented the findings of the study he and his colleagues completed on resident-to-staff aggression. They found that resident-to-staff aggression, including verbal, physical, and sexual aggression, was extremely common, with more than 15 percent of residents exhibiting such aggression within the previous 2-week period. Residents demonstrating resident-to-staff aggression were more likely to be white, require more assistance with activities of daily living, and have affective and behavioral disturbances.

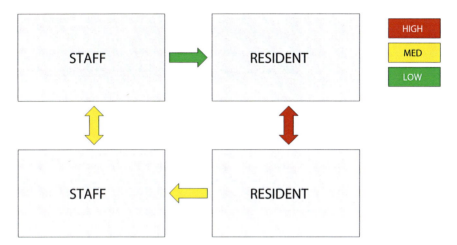

FIGURE 2-1 Actual (versus potential) harm to the largest number of residents.
SOURCE: Lachs, 2013.

Lachs defined resident-to-resident elder mistreatment as "negative and aggressive physical, sexual, or verbal interactions between long-term care residents that would likely be construed as unwelcome by the recipient in a community setting, and that have high potential to cause physical or psychological distress." In terms of prevalence estimations, measuring resident-to-resident violence is extremely challenging. Lachs noted that for domestic violence, a large amount of the data is collected through self-reporting; however, in nursing home settings, rates of cognitive impairment are so high that self-reporting can result in high levels of false positives and false negatives. Despite the challenges of measuring resident-to-resident aggression within institutions, Lachs suggested that with innovative methods and a research agenda, it can be done. Currently, a National Institute on Aging–funded study of resident-to-resident elder mistreatment in 10 facilities is employing methodology to try to ascertain prevalence rates and identify resident, facility, and contextual correlates. The study is triangulating case findings from multiple sources, including (1) a culturally validated instrument administered to residents and primary certified nursing assistants; (2) incident reports; and (3) "shift coupons," a novel method adapted for staff identification of resident-to-resident mistreatment in real time.

Workshop speaker Pamela Teaster from the University of Kentucky commented that the evidence so far indicates that abuse occurs more predominantly in the community setting and more dominantly by family and friends than other individuals, but the field still has much to do to understand the nuances of types of abuse. She remarked, "Those types of individuals who may be the offenders, the abusers, the perpetrators, can also be spouses, can also be other intimate partners, can also be carers, can also be paid, can also be providing volunteer services; all those individuals in community settings or in facility settings can be potential victims and can be potential abusers."

COGNITIVE IMPAIRMENT

As was recognized in discussions about the settings in which abuse occurs, cognitive impairment is a unique challenge in elder abuse. Several speakers commented that, when addressing elder abuse, distinction should be made between cognitive impairment and non-cognitive impairment, as the remedies will be different. Acierno suggested that abuse against non-cognitively impaired older adults is violence against an independent adult by an independent adult, and thus should be perceived as domestic violence. In domestic violence, the intervention is very different than in child abuse, in which a non-independent, non-empowered individual is being abused by an independent, empowered individual.

Recognizing that cognitive impairment is and will be a major problem that has to be addressed in the field of elder abuse, workshop speaker Jason Karlawish from the University of Pennsylvania suggested two important ways in which cognitive impairment and elder abuse intersect. First, cognitive impairment has been recognized as a problem and national attention is being paid to addressing it as a disease-based problem. One of the first signs of cognitive impairment is the inability to manage finances, which also is one of the risk factors for being a victim of elder abuse and exploitation. The more elder abuse awareness and prevention is linked to a disease-based mandate that has policy makers' attention, such as cognitive impairment, the more progress can be made. Second, Karlawish noted that the field of cognitive impairment deals with biological, pathological, clinical, and ethical issues, including ethical issues on elder abuse.

Phillips commented that, in many developing countries, less than 1 percent of the seriously disabled elderly are in institutions. Thus, while elder abuse often is characterized by the setting, either in the community or in an institution, such a characterization does not necessarily distinguish between those who are cognitively impaired and those who are non-cognitively impaired. Phillips further elaborated that there are levels of cognitive impairment to consider: those who are severely demented and therefore incapable of expressing their own desires, and those who are mildly demented and have some degree of capacity. In addition, within institutions, there are individuals with physical illness who are not necessarily cognitively impaired. Therefore, one way to consider characterizing elder abuse and its remedies could be to think of a matrix with six categories:

the three levels of cognitive impairment and in the setting of either the community or the institutions. Workshop speaker Gil Livingston from the University College of London agreed with this point. She noted that types of elder abuse, whether occurring in the home or in institutions or to someone who is cognitively intact or not, are very different and there will not be a one-size-fits-all solution.

NEGLECT AND SELF-NEGLECT

Speaker and planning committee member Terry Fulmer from Northeastern University stressed that although neglect and self-neglect are often grouped with other forms of elder abuse, there is a need to consistently tease out what is neglect versus abuse because of the unique challenges associated with both neglect and self-neglect. Based on the data she has reviewed, Fulmer conservatively estimated that 4 percent of elders experience neglect; however, she suggested that, based on the difficulties associated with prevalence studies for elder neglect, the rate is likely much higher.

Rather than being defined by the infliction of injury and suffering, neglect is a failure to provide services necessary to maintain physical and mental health. According to the 2003 National Research Council (NRC) report *Elder Mistreatment*, neglect is defined as "an omission by responsible caregivers that constitutes 'neglect' under applicable federal or state law" (NRC, 2003, p. 39). The National Center on Elder Abuse defines neglect as "refusal or failure by those responsible to provide food, shelter, health care or protection for a vulnerable elder" (National Center on Elder Abuse, 2013).

Self-neglect was defined in the 2003 NRC report as "failure of individual to provide essential services for self as result of mental or physical inability" (NRC, 2003, p. 37). Workshop speaker Carmel Dyer from the University of Texas presented a model that she and her colleagues published in 2007 that demonstrates the risk factors for elder self-neglect. As shown in the model, self-neglect begins with neurodegenerative and mental health issues, and then executive dysfunction sets in, followed by impairment in activities of daily living. When coupled with inadequate support services due to lack of capacity for self-care and self-protection, or because of extrinsic issues like poverty access or lack of social support, self-neglect can result. Current research has provided an evidence base for the model.

Workshop speaker Kathleen Quinn from the National Adult Protective Services Association noted that issues of caregiver neglect are often complicated when a spouse is providing the care. For example, she suggested there are situations where a 100-pound, 80-year-old woman with osteoporosis is trying to care for her 175-pound husband who had a stroke. She does not want to be separated from him, she wants to care for him, she does her best, but she cannot provide the care.

The question of an individual's right to self-neglect was brought up by several speakers, acknowledging that the decision to self-neglect is related to the right to self-determination. Quinn noted that the Adult Protective Services (APS) code of ethics is based on self-determination, an adults' right to make their own decisions and refuse intervention if they choose. However, she noted that the question always comes down to "Can they make those decisions?" and then "Who decides?"

Dong asked, "How do we determine the continuity of self-neglect and neglect? Because somebody is living by themselves? Their family is upstairs? At a point where do we determine there is a caregiving responsibility?" He suggested that within certain cultures, such as Chinese culture, there is an assumption of caregiving responsibility on family members regardless if they live in the same house or have moved away. Quinn responded that, in terms of APS, within the United States each state has different definitions for what constitutes neglect. In Illinois, where she worked, the definition is that once somebody undertakes care, they cannot stop providing care in an irresponsible manner. Dyer reported that, based on a survey of APS workers in Houston, they found that APS workers were differentiating between neglect and self-neglect based on whether someone else was living in the house because clinically there is little difference. Fulmer agreed, but stressed that for the purpose of building the evidence and moving the field forward, decisions on definitions need to be made rather than delaying the research.

CONCEPTUALIZING ELDER ABUSE

No overarching theory or conceptual framework exists for elder abuse, and workshop speakers debated the value in developing one and potentially "borrowing" concepts from existing theoretical frameworks.

Workshop speaker Pamela Teaster from the University of Kentucky presented several frameworks that have been applied to elder abuse or have the potential to be applicable to elder abuse; however, she acknowledged that each of them have deficits (see Table 2-1). Rather than suggesting a particular theory to be applied to elder abuse, Teaster proposed several overarching characteristics that any theoretical conceptualization of elder abuse should include transdisciplinarity, global context, community versus institutional setting, levels of cognitive impairment, balancing individual rights with safety, and inclusion of both upstream and downstream issues.

Greenlee suggested that part of the success in the work of domestic violence has been the critical support and training to include law enforcement. Elder abuse is a crime and whatever theoretical framework is developed, it needs to be translatable to law enforcement, prosecutors, and judges so that

TABLE 2-1 Conceptual Frameworks and Perspective on Their Applicability to Elder Abuse

Framework	Perspective on Applicability to Elder Abuse
Ecological Model (Bronfenbrenner, 1979)	• Originally conceptualized for children • Provides a multilevel, nested systems approach to considering the problem • Highlights the importance of "levels" or layers of thinking • Attaches responsibility/responsivity to micro through macrosystems • Systems are not intersecting, but rather nested • Difficult to measure or consider all of these when conducting research or designing interventions • Idea of time "Chronosystem" is difficult to apply
Sociocultural Model (NRC, 2003)	• Specifically designed to explain elder mistreatment • Like the Ecological Model, considers a variety of contributors to mistreatment • Builds on elders in relationship with others • Considers dynamics of power, exchange, and inequality • Includes outcomes • Issue of the "trusted other" • Does not include self-neglect • Does not address "time" • Needs deeper consideration of characteristics of the abuser
Cycle of Violence Theory (Walker, 1979)	• Derived from the domestic violence literature • Situational and short term • Easily comprehensible to laypersons • Not everyone who commits elder abuse was reared in a home in which violence took place • Could excuse the perpetrator from culpability • Inconsistent support for this theory
Lifecourse Perspective (Kuh and Ben-Shlomo, 1997)	• Provides context for action and intervention • Multiple ways to apply • "Not a theory" conundrum • Misapplication of central tendency • Confounding social change and social forces • Neglects intercohort variability • Confuses time with change • Making choices becomes a "problem"

SOURCE: Presented by Pamela Teaster, University of Kentucky.

it supports the understanding of elder abuse as a criminal activity. She also commented on the applicability of the public health model to elder abuse. Greenlee noted that as a lawyer by training and as a public servant, she has struggled with applying the public health structure and the categorization of primary, secondary, and tertiary prevention to elder abuse because of ageism. Articulating primary prevention for older people is very hard to do. She posited putting the model on its head with tertiary first and then secondary and then primary, because primary is such a struggle. Greenlee suggested that if a framework can be developed that achieves these objectives, of overcoming ageism and being inclusive of law enforcement, she could work with any structure that is developed.

Several workshop speakers noted the contagious nature of elder abuse, both within a setting and across the lifespan.[1] Lachs spoke of cultures of violence and suggested that the ecological model, which considers factors at the individual, family, community, and societal levels and how they influence each other, could be a useful model for elder abuse. He added that the ecologic model of violence has been recognized as valid and highly suitable for developing intervention. Several speakers noted that many victims of elder abuse experienced other forms of violence earlier in life (Dong, 2013). Considering earlier exposures to violence, the lifecourse perspective could be a valuable framework for conceptualizing elder abuse. Workshop planning committee and Forum co-chair Jacquelyn Campbell suggested that some frameworks are useful for prevention by identifying risk factors, while others are useful for developing interventions.

ISSUES WITH PREVALENCE STUDIES

Livingston pointed out that the problem of knowing who to ask about elder abuse makes measuring difficult. Some researchers ask older adults themselves, while others rely on third-party assessments by family members or professionals, or data from APS or the police. Lachs raised the difficulty of getting prevalence estimates for neglect because through typical modes of collecting prevalence data—including screening in health care settings—individuals, particularly those with cognitive impairments, are largely excluded. He suggested a need for global mapping and novel high-risk methodology to get community-based prevalence estimates. Wallace stressed the need to look at multiple sources to get a better picture of what is going on in the community and suggested a need for multiple modes of

---

[1] For more information, see Dong, X. 2012. *Elder abuse and the contagion of violence*, Discussion Paper, Institute of Medicine, Washington, DC. http://iom.edu/Global/Perspectives/2012/ElderAbuse.aspx (accessed October 14, 2013).

data collection, as prevalence surveys by themselves are important but not sufficient.

> **Key Messages Raised by Individual Speakers**
>
> - There is a high prevalence of elder abuse in community-residing elders, primarily domestic violence (Acierno, Teaster).
> - Conceptualizations and definitions of elder abuse need to be culturally relevant (Chang, Dong, Jervis, Mouton, Yan).
> - The distinction between elder neglect and self-neglect often is not easy to determine and is defined differently by institutions and by communities (Dyer, Fulmer, Quinn).
> - No overarching conceptual framework for elder abuse exists (Teaster).

REFERENCES

Acierno, R., M. A. Hernandez, A. B. Amstadter, H. S. Resnick, K. Steve, W. Muzzy, and D. G. Kilpatrick. 2010. Prevalence and correlates of emotional, physical, sexual, and financial abuse and potential neglect in the United States: The National Elder Mistreatment Study. *American Journal of Public Health* 100(2):292-297.

Bronfenbrenner, U. 1979. *The ecology of human development: Experiments by nature and design.* Cambridge, MA: Harvard University Press.

CDC (Centers for Disease Control and Prevention). 2013. *Elder abuse: Definitions.* http://www.cdc.gov/violenceprevention/elderabuse/definitions.html (accessed September 13, 2013).

Dong, X. 2013. *The pine report.* Chicago, IL: Rush Institute for Health Aging, Rush University Medical Center.

Kuh, D., and Y. Ben-Shlomo. 1997. *A life course approach to chronic disease epidemiology.* New York: Oxford Univeristy Press.

National Center on Elder Abuse. 2013. *Types of abuse.* http://www.ncea.aoa.gov/FAQ/Type_Abuse (accessed April 15, 2013).

NRC (National Research Council). 2003. *Elder mistreatment: Abuse, neglect, and exploitation in an aging America.* Washington, DC: The National Academies Press.

Walker, L. 1979. *The battered woman.* New York: Harper and Row.

3

Risk Factors and Health Outcomes

The prevalence of abuse and the context in which it occurs provide an important but incomplete picture of the overall burden of elder abuse. As presented by Robert Wallace from the University of Iowa and XinQi Dong from the Rush Institute for Healthy Aging, factors have been identified that are associated with an increased risk for elder abuse, and adverse health outcomes have been shown to be associated with occurrences of abuse. Understanding these risk factors and health outcomes could help demonstrate the magnitude of elder abuse and opportunities for prevention.

RISK FACTORS

Identifying and understanding factors that are associated with both predicting and protecting from occurrences of elder abuse is key to determining how to prevent abuse, particularly through primary prevention. Planning committee member Jeffrey Hall from the Centers for Disease Control and Prevention elaborated: "When we know what factors combined make perpetration more or less likely and when we understand what processes and conditions may create vulnerabilities, we first can act meaningfully and decisively to protect and promote the health of older adults, and, secondly, we can gain insights on the kinds and configurations of strategies that prevent further abuse, neglect, or exploitation by a variety of different perpetrator categories that we know exist." Hall also noted that, within the context of the ecological framework, consideration needs to be given to how risk factors originate in different levels of social interaction—between individuals,

TABLE 3-1 Risk Factors for Elder Mistreatment and Being a Perpetrator

Risk Factors for Elder Mistreatment	Risk Factors for Being a Perpetrator[a]

• Victim dependency/vulnerability
  o Poor health; disability/functional impairment; poor personal defenses; poverty; possibly dementing illnesses (responses to behavior)
• Gender—women
• Abuser dependency/deviance
  o Alcohol and drug abuse; mental illness; poor employment record
• Social isolation
  o Abuse undetected; lack of social support to buffer stress
• Living arrangements
  o Shared living arrangements; greater opportunity for tension and conflict; long-term care facilities
• Resources to exploit
	• Alcohol and substance abuse
	• Mental health problems: depression/personality disorder; behavioral problems; caregiver burnout, inexperience
	• Poor interpersonal relationships; premorbid relations
	• Current marital, family conflict
	• Lack of empathy, understanding of care needs and issues
	• Financially dependent on victim

[a] Abusive Caregiver Characteristics (Reis and Nahmiash, 1998).
SOURCE: Presented by Robert Wallace, University of Iowa.

within relationships and communities, and in the social environments that surround them. It is also important to explore and understand how such influences operate in different settings and cultural contexts.

Workshop speaker Robert Wallace from the University of Iowa acknowledged that there is a range of risk factors for both perpetrating and being a victim of elder mistreatment—some that are rather straightforward and others that are complicated to both identify and address (see Table 3-1). He noted that these known risk factors have been derived mostly from case-control studies; however, prospective studies are needed to better describe the range of risk factors and be able to make significant progress toward prevention. Workshop speaker Ron Acierno from the University of South Carolina noted that, while elder mistreatment perpetrated by strangers and caregivers is different, there are risk factors that overlap, and understanding the overlap is important for designing effective interventions.

Possible New Approaches to Addressing Elder Mistreatment Risk Factors and Prevention

Wallace noted several newer approaches to addressing elder mistreatment risk factors and prevention that have the potential to move the field forward:

- Considering aging in society through the lenses of ageism, human rights, larger social and cultural attitudes, going beyond interpersonal relations, and social exchanges and transactions.
- Geographic context and information through violent crime mapping.
- Life course experience and victimization: possible role for adverse childhood experiences.
- Possible genetic effects.
- Development of potential screening "biomarkers."
- Role of forensic science.
- Elder monitoring and telemedicine.

Potential Areas for Further Research

The following section of the report outlines several areas in which further research on specific factors was suggested by workshop speakers.

Social Support

Several workshop speakers suggested that increasing social support through community integration could help protect vulnerable adults from elder abuse. For example, better access to public transportation was discussed as a potential avenue for decreasing isolation. However, Acierno pointed out that research is needed to understand what types of social support are effective for preventing elder abuse and how they can be amplified, as well as which types are not effective, or possibly even harmful. Agnes Tiwari from the University of Hong Kong expanded on this point by commenting that, within the field of domestic violence prevention, which has been grappling with the issue of social support for years, one thing that has been learned is that even though the same principles may apply, different people need different social support. For instance, some people may prefer to have family members or friends involved in an intervention, while others might prefer that the people they know are not involved. The context in which the abuse or potential abuse occurs matters and the role of social support as a protective factor for elder abuse prevention needs to be better understood.

Substance Abuse

Evidence suggests a relationship between substance abuse and violence, both in victimization and perpetration, and some limited research suggesting a relationship between substance abuse and elder abuse specifically (Bushman and Cooper, 1990; Dolan, 1999; Sripada et al., 2011; Jogerst et al., 2012). Wallace noted that alcoholism often does not start in late life, but rather is a factor that may have been ongoing across a lifetime that has results in complicated long-term social interactions. Several speakers agreed that there is need for more research on the relationship between substance abuse and elder abuse, and alcohol abuse and elder abuse.

Life Course Perspective

Wallace asked, "When does elder mistreatment begin?" He referenced some work that has been done in other areas of violence and abuse, such as violence against women, that links previous victimization with future victimization or perpetration. He suggested that researchers should be asking questions about previous experiences of violence to older adults as well, so the lifecourse perspective and early childhood adverse-experience effects on elder abuse can be better understood as a potential risk factor. Workshop speaker E-Shien Chang from the Rush Institute on Healthy Aging noted that from the data from the Pine Report, one-third of the victims who screened positive for elder abuse had experienced other types of abuse earlier in life before the age of 60 (Dong, 2013).

Depression

Forum member Michael Phillips from the Shanghai Jiao Tao Medical School commented on the relationship between depression and elder abuse, particularly neglect and self-neglect. Depression can be a factor contributing to one's decision to self-neglect; also, neglect can further exacerbate depression, creating a vicious cycle. The extent of depression in mistreated older adults is not known and, if left untreated, can lead to more abuse and other types of mistreatment. Phillips also noted that depression is treatable and that fact should not be overlooked, even in older adults. He suggested that more research should be pursued on the relationship between elder abuse and depression.

HEALTH OUTCOMES

Hall asked, "Why focus on the aftermath of the abuse?" He noted that in assessing the magnitude and effect of elder abuse, the prevalence and incidence data only reveal a small portion of the public health burden of this problem. Abuse, neglect, and exploitation adversely affect physical and mental capacity and impairments, social positions, and structures. In addition, they may exacerbate existing health conditions that already affect an older person's well-being and can render disease and prevention promotion activities ineffective or unrealistic. Abuse may place older adults on health trajectories where they will die earlier than older adults with no history of elder abuse victimization (Lachs et al., 1998).

Workshop planning committee co-chair and Forum member XinQi Dong from the Rush Institute for Healthy Aging presented an overview of adverse health outcomes of elder abuse. Data in this area was first presented in 1998 with the New Haven cohort study of residence that matched data to Adult Protective Services and demonstrated an independent relationship between elder abuse and mortality (Lachs et al., 1998). In the same cohort, the relationship with the long-term care placement was shown as well. Some of the later work by Margaret Baker and colleagues (2009) suggested that perhaps there was not as strong a link with mortality as previously thought. The Chicago Healthy Aging Project (CHAP), a 14-year prospective population-based study conducted in Chicago of nearly 10,000 community-dwelling older adults, has produced data showing the association between elder abuse and mortality, as well as associations with other health outcomes and indicators of health outcomes. Dong presented findings from the CHAP, which are summarized in Table 3-2.

Despite the contributions from the research that has been done to date, Acierno noted that still very little is known about elder abuse association with health outcomes, such as depression, stress, and other mental health consequences. More research is needed to better understand the relationship between elder abuse and a wider range of health outcomes.

TABLE 3-2 Summary of Chicago Healthy Aging Project (CHAP) Findings

Elder abuse and mortality	The data from the CHAP study has shown 5.9 deaths per 100 for those without elder abuse and 18.3 per 100 people with elder abuse. Mortality risk was higher among those with greater cognitive and functional impairment. Cardiovascular-related mortality risk was particularly high. Because the study was done over 14 years, the health of the participants changed over time and that was taken into consideration (Dong et al., 2009).
Elder self-neglect and mortality	The CHAP study data have shown reported elder self-neglect was associated with a significantly increased risk of 1-year mortality (Dong et al., 2009). The CHAP study data also have shown that, persisting over time, the impact of self-neglect on mortality was significantly stronger in black than in white older adults (Dong et al., 2011c).

TABLE 3-2 Continued

Elder self-neglect and emergency department (ED) use	Elder self-neglect is associated with increased rate of ED use and greater self-neglect severity is associated with greater increase in ED use (Dong et al., 2011b).
Elder abuse and mortality: psychosocial well-being	Mortality risk associated with elder abuse was most prominent among those with highest levels of depressive symptoms and lowest levels of social network and social engagement (Dong et al., 2011a).
Elder self-neglect and hospitalization	Elder self-neglect is associated with higher rate of hospitalization. This relationship was not moderated by medical comorbidities or cognitive or physical function (Dong et al., 2012; Dong and Simon, 2013d).
Elder self-neglect and hospice use	Elder self-neglect is associated with increased risk of hospice use, shorter length of stay in hospice care, and shorter time from hospice admission to death (Dong and Simon, 2013c).
Elder self-neglect and elder abuse	Elder self-neglect reporting is associated with increased risk for subsequent elder abuse reporting to social services agency (Dong et al., 2013).
Elder abuse and ED use	Elder abuse was associated with increased rates of ED use, and specific subtypes of elder abuse had differential association with increased rate of ED use (Dong and Simon, 2013a).
Elder abuse and hospitalization	Elder abuse was associated with increased rates of hospitalization (Dong and Simon, 2013d).
Elder abuse and skilled nursing facility (SNF) admissions	Elder abuse was associated with increased rates of admission to SNF. Specific subtypes of elder abuse had a differential association with an increased rate of admission to SNF (Dong and Simon, 2013b).

REFERENCES

Baker, M. W., A. Z. LaCroix, C. Wu, B. B. Cochrane, R. Wallace, and N. F. Woods. 2009. Mortality risk associated with physical and verbal abuse in women aged 50 to 79. *Journal of the American Geriatrics Society* 57(10):1799-1809.

Bushman, B. J., and H. M. Cooper. 1990. Effects of alcohol on human-aggression—an integrative research review. *Psychological Bulletin* 107(3):341-354.

Dolan, V. F. 1999. Risk factors for elder abuse. *Journal of Insurance Medicine* 31(1):13-20.

Dong, X. 2013. *The pine report*. Chicago, IL: Rush Institute for Health Aging, Rush University Medical Center.

Dong, X., and M. A. Simon. 2013a. Association between elder abuse and use of ED: Findings from the Chicago Health and Aging Project. *The American Journal of Emergency Medicine* 31(4):693-698.

Dong, X., and M. A. Simon. 2013b. Association between reported elder abuse and rates of admission to skilled nursing facilities: Findings from a longitudinal population-based cohort study. *Gerontology* 59(5):464-472.

Dong, X., and M. A. Simon. 2013c. Association between elder self-neglect and hospice utilization in a community population. *Archives of Gerontology and Geriatrics* 56(1):192-198.

Dong, X., and M. A. Simon. 2013d. Elder abuse as a risk factor for hospitalization in older persons. *JAMA Internal Medicine* 173(10):911-917.

Dong, X., M. Simon, C. Mendes de Leon, T. Fulmer, T. Beck, L. Hebert, C. Dyer, G. Paveza, and D. Evans. 2009. Elder self-neglect and abuse and mortality risk in a community-dwelling population. *Journal of the American Medical Association* 302(5):517-526.

Dong, X. Q., M. A. Simon, T. T. Beck, C. Farran, J. J. McCann, C. F. M. de Leon, E. Laumann, and D. A. Evans. 2011a. Elder abuse and mortality: The role of psychological and social wellbeing. *Gerontology* 57(6):549-558.

Dong, X., M. A. Simon, and D. A. Evans. 2011b. Prospective study of the elder self-neglect and emergency department use in a community population. *American Journal of Emergency Medicine* 30:553-556.

Dong, X. Q., M. A. Simon, T. Fulmer, C. F. Mendes de Leon, L. E. Hebert, T. Beck, P. A. Scherr, and D. A. Evans. 2011c. A prospective population-based study of differences in elder self-neglect and mortality between black and white older adults. *Journals of Gerontology Series A-Biological Sciences and Medical Sciences* 66(6):695-704.

Dong, X., M. A. Simon, and D. Evans. 2012. Elder self-neglect and hospitalization: Findings from the Chicago health and aging project. *Journal of the American Geriatrics Society* 60(2):202-209.

Dong, X., M. A. Simon, and D. Evans. 2013. Elder self-neglect is associated with increased risk for elder abuse in a community-dwelling population: Findings from the Chicago Health and Aging Project. *Journal of Aging and Health* 25(1):80-96.

Jogerst, G. J., J. M. Daly, L. J. Galloway, S. Zheng, and Y. Xu. 2012. Substance abuse associated with elder abuse in the United States. *American Journal of Drug & Alcohol Abuse* 38(1):63-69.

Lachs, M. S., C. S. Williams, S. O'Brien, K. A. Pillemer, and M. E. Charlson. 1998. The mortality of elder mistreatment. *Journal of the American Medical Association* 280(5):428-432.

Reis, M., and D. Nahmiash. 1998. Validation of the indicators of abuse (IOA) screen. *Gerontologist* 38:471-480.

Sripada, C. S., M. Angstadt, P. McNamara, A. C. King, and K. L. Phan. 2011. Effects of alcohol on brain responses to social signals of threat in humans. *NeuroImage* 55(1):371-380.

4

Ethical Considerations

What are the ethical goals of elder abuse prevention? What are the ethical challenges and issues in preventing and intervening in abuse and neglect? Workshop panelists discussed these issues in the context of providing care and services, and opportunities for prevention.

Workshop speaker Susan Lynch from the Department of Justice suggested that the goals of elder abuse prevention are to prevent unnecessary suffering, maintain autonomy, and maintain quality of life. Within this context, she laid out four principles to consider in elder abuse prevention:

1. Autonomy is the right to self-determination, independence, and freedom. Autonomy expresses the concept that professionals have a duty to treat the person according to the person's desires, within the bounds of accepted treatment, and to protect the individual's confidentiality.
2. Justice is the obligation to be fair to all people.
3. Beneficence requires that health care providers do good for individuals under their care by understanding the individual from a holistic perspective that includes the individual's beliefs, feelings, and wishes as well as those of the individual's family and significant others.
4. Nonmaleficence is the requirement that health care providers do no harm to their patients and that they protect their patients from harm.

In making decisions on which ethical issues to focus its resources, Lynch noted that the Department of Justice, with funding support from the Department of Health and Human Services, developed a concept map of the field of elder abuse. They started the process by inviting 750 professionals from the field to respond to this statement: "To understand, prevent, identify, or respond to elder abuse, to collect or exhortation we need." The feedback from this process was used to generate ideas that were categorized and rated for feasibility and importance. Through this process, the key ethical issues that were identified were brain health and function, elder abuse reporting, provisions under the Health Insurance Portability and Accountability Act of 1996 (HIPAA), and long-term care quality and abuse prevention.

BRAIN HEALTH AND FUNCTION: DECISION-MAKING CAPACITY AND COMPETENCY

Within the area of brain health and function, the primary concern is an individual's decision-making capacity and competency. Lynch defined decision-making capacity as the ability to understand the nature and consequences of different options, to make choices among those options, and to communicate that choice. Decision-making capacity is required in order to give informed consent. Such capacity may fluctuate over time, given the state of health of the individual as well as the particular issue.

Another issue related to brain function and health is the notion of competency. Competency is defined legally and determines if an individual is fit and qualified to give testimony or executive a legal document. In the United States, the law presumes all adults are competent and have decision-making capacities to make health decisions unless deemed otherwise in court. Lynch discussed ethical issues within the legal system about the capacity of a vulnerable adult to testify in an elder abuse case. She noted that a lack of competency could be used as a defense litigation strategy to preclude testimony from victims or witnesses of abuse.

Lynch also discussed ethical issues around informed consent in research studies and the decisional capacity of older adults. She noted that, after being given information, a person gives informed consent when he or she can make a choice, understand and appreciate the issues, rationally manipulate information, and make a stable and coherent decision. Several considerations for what may impede an older adult's ability to give informed consent are sensory deficits, impaired ability to ask questions, and values and beliefs about making health care choices.

Assessing Capacity

Workshop speaker Jason Karlawish from the University of Pennsylvania expanded on the issue of assessing decisional capacity. Both the theory and practice of capacity assessment have made substantial progress in developing a coherent set of concepts and practices that are legally and ethically acceptable. Karlawish has studied the history of the concepts of decisional capacity and competency since the 1960s, and much of the debate about capacity and competency has centered on different meanings being applied to the same words or the same word being used with different meanings. However, he believes the field has arrived at a reasonable place with legally and ethically acceptable concepts. Decisional capacity is the continuum of decision-making abilities: choice, understanding, appreciation, and reasoning. Assessments of adequate capacity for decision making are used to make judgments of competency.

Karlawish discussed in detail financial capacity, which is defined as "the ability to manage money and financial assets in ways that meet a person's needs and which are consistent with his or her values and self-interest" (Marson et al., 2011). Karlawish suggested that financial capacity is a multidimensional construct that consists of four elements: (1) having basic monetary skills, (2) carrying out cash transactions, (3) managing a checkbook and bank statement, and (4) exercising financial judgment. Karlawish noted that this specific kind of capacity can be thought of not as a "decisional capacity," but as an activity of daily living akin to cooking, shopping, or cleaning. He suggested there should be an instrument for assessing financial capacity that is standard practice for Adult Protective Services (APS) workers.

Assessment for the Capacity for Everyday Decision Making

Karlawish and his colleagues have developed an instrument called the assessment for the capacity for everyday decision making (ACED), which helps providers answer the question "are patients who refuse interventions to help them manage their IADL [instrumental activity of daily living] disabilities capable of making this decision?" (Lai and Karlawish, 2007). Through validation of the tool, they found that a substantial number of older adults with cognitive impairments caused by Alzheimer's or its variants, from very mild to moderate severity, could all express a choice; that is, all of them could tell you what they would want or not want. Most of them could reason through that choice; that is, they could give you consequences. However, they exhibited problems with understanding the information, such as what their checkbook is for or how cooking works. He noted that in many capacity cases there are two distinct questions: Can someone

	Able to perform IADL?	
	YES	NO
Able to decide how to manage IADL impairment — YES	living independently	dependent and ok
Able to decide how to manage IADL impairment — NO	NA	(dependent and not OK)

FIGURE 4-1 Ethical considerations in research and care.
NOTE: IADL = instrumental activity of daily living.
SOURCE: Karlawish, 2013.

independently perform an IADL? and When presented solutions to manage a problem performing an IADL, can the person use those solutions to solve the problem? These are two separate decisions, and an individual could be capable of doing one, but not the other. Karlawish presented a two-by-two matrix that pairs assessing the ability to perform IADL with the ability to decide how to manage IADL impairment (see Figure 4-1).

These abilities are both issues of capacity—one ability is about doing a task and the other is about making a decision on how best to manage a problem with that task. Karlawish suggested that the field is at a point of being able to train individuals in performing this assessment so ethical decisions can be made about an individual's ability to perform an IADL and, if they are impaired, their ability to make a decision about how to manage that impairment. Education on and dissemination of tools for assessment are needed for those in the field, such as APS workers, who are expected to assess these capacities on a regular basis.

ELDER ABUSE REPORTING

Lynch discussed ethical considerations as well as barriers for elder abuse reporting, which has led to underreporting. Focusing on provider issues, she noted that, most states have mandatory reporting requirements for both abuse and neglect that apply to medical professionals, health care providers, mental health counselors, service providers, and government agents who come in contact with the elderly. However, to overcome some of the barriers to reporting, Lynch suggested that providers will need at least:

(1) a common definition of what abuse is and the different types of abuse, (2) awareness of reporting laws, and (3) knowledge and understanding of the next steps after reporting.

HIPAA

Lynch noted that HIPAA, which was created to protect medical information, has been perceived as a barrier to information sharing on elder abuse issues between emergency medical services and prosecutors; between hospitals and prosecutors; and among emergency medical services, hospitals, and APS. However, there are several exceptions to HIPAA that allow covered entities to provide protected health information to law enforcement and social service agencies. Lynch said a better public education effort is needed to explain these exceptions. Lynch identified several of these exceptions:

- Required by law/mandatory reporting laws: A covered entity may disclose protected health information to law enforcement officials if it is required to do so by law. An example would be a state law mandating the reporting of certain wounds or other physical injuries.
- Victims of a crime: Health care entities may also provide law enforcement officials with an individual's protected health information if the individual is a suspected victim of a crime. In such cases, covered entities can only disclose information if (1) the individual agrees to disclosure, or (2) the covered entity cannot obtain the individual's agreement because of incapacity or an emergency.
- Victims of abuse, neglect, or domestic violence: A covered entity that believes an individual has been the victim of abuse may disclose the individual's protected health information to a government agency that is authorized by law to receive reports of abuse, neglect, or domestic violence.

LONG-TERM CARE

Lynch outlined several legal remedies for issues of elder abuse in long-term care facilities. Cases can be brought through the False Claims Act (FCA), under which individuals who knowingly file false claims for Medicare or Medicaid payments can be liable for damages and penalties. Through FCA, providers who render substandard or no care that may harm the patient and bill Medicare or Medicaid can be pursued. Cases have been brought against nursing facilities, assisted living facilities, psychiatric and acute care hospitals, and group homes.

MOVING FORWARD

The panelists offered suggestions for priority issues in the area of ethical considerations to move the field forward. Lynch suggested there is a need for more evidence and, when appropriate, more prosecution of elder abuse cases. Noting the availability of assessment tools, Karlawish suggested that education on and dissemination of tools for assessment are needed for professionals in the field, such as APS workers, who are expected to assess decisional capacity on a regular basis. Speaker Sidney Stahl suggested there is an ethical imperative for more research and research funding, specifically in the areas of APS interventions and primary and secondary prevention.

REFERENCES

Karlawish, J. 2013. *Elder abuse and neglect: Ethical consideration in research and care.* Presented at Elder Abuse and Its Prevention: A Workshop. Institute of Medicine, Washington, DC, April 17.

Lai, J. M., and J. Karlawish. 2007. Assessing the capacity to make everyday decisions: A guide for clinicians and an agenda for future research. *American Journal of Geriatric Psychiatry* 15(2):101-111.

Marson, D. C., K. Hebert, and A. C. Solomon. 2011. Assessing civil competencies in older adults with dementia: Consent capacity, financial capacity, and testamentary capacity. In *Forensic neuropsychology: A scientific approach*, edited by G. J. Larrabee (2nd ed.). New York: Oxford University Press. Pp. 401-437.

5

Screening and Prevention

While the previous chapters have underscored the magnitude and burden of elder abuse and unique challenges that they present, this chapter focuses on applying what is known toward detecting and preventing abuse. Existing tools and models for screening and intervention are presented, along with discussions on increasing the effectiveness of ongoing efforts and opportunities for new interventions.

SCREENING

Screening tools have been developed for the detection of multiple forms of violence, including intimate partner violence, child abuse, and elder abuse. The effectiveness of such tools has been debated. Although the U.S. Preventive Services Task Force recommends that clinicians screen women for intimate partner violence, it has concluded that the current evidence for elder abuse and neglect screening is insufficient to assess its potential benefits or harm.[1] Although the existing evidence is limited, considering the association between elder abuse and adverse health outcomes and the association of elder abuse with increased health services use, efforts are being made to develop and assess screening tools in multiple settings and grow the evidence base on their effectiveness. Workshop panelists presented some of these current efforts as well as challenges and opportunities for moving elder abuse screening and detection forward. A detailed overview of both

---

[1] See http://www.uspreventiveservicestaskforce.org/uspstf/uspsipv.htm.

screening tools and issues presented at the workshop are included in Part II of this report (see *McMullen et al.*). Below is a brief summary.

Workshop planning committee member Tara McMullen and speaker Kimberly Schwartz from the Centers for Medicare & Medicaid Services (CMS) presented the agency's work in the areas of measuring and assessing elder abuse. CMS began this work because of the recognized lack of universal agreement on how to measure all aspects of elder maltreatment. One of the challenges CMS has identified with its current measure, the Elder Maltreatment Screen and Follow-up Plan, is that it seldom is reported by eligible providers, and CMS wants to increase the feasibility and reporting of its measure.

Workshop speaker Mark Yaffe from McGill University presented the Elder Abuse Suspicion Index (EASI), which is administered by family physicians in primary care settings. The EASI tool is intended to generate suspicion about the presence of mistreatment or neglect sufficient to justify further discussion of the issue between doctor and patient, or patient referral to a community expert in elder abuse for in-depth evaluation. Yaffe commented that family physicians are well positioned to detect elder abuse for several reasons: They may be the only people outside of family who regularly see some older adults. Often there is an established trust in a doctor–patient relationship, and trust in theory helps to promote disclosure; most patients are accustomed to doctors asking direct questions about sensitive topics, and the physical exam is an opportunity to look for abnormal lab findings and unexplained deterioration. Yaffe discussed several barriers to elder abuse screening in primary care settings: lack of awareness of elder abuse and its association with higher mortality rates, lack of knowledge of how to identify it, previous absence of screening detection tools that were appropriate for use in a doctor's office, considerations about ethical and confidentiality issues, disbelief that detection will lead to a solution, ageism, concerns about legal issues, and confusing guidelines.

Yaffe also suggested that the focus of a family doctor's approach should be evidence informed and patient centered. Forum member Brigid McCaw from Kaiser Permanente agreed that screening tools need to focus on patient centeredness, as well as facilitating clinician behavior change. As the implementers, physicians need to see the value in screening so that the tools will be used more often. Schwartz noted that a focus of CMS's work on elder abuse measurement is to make it more patient centered and driven more toward an outcome-based versus a process-based measure. Workshop speaker Susan Lynch from the Department of Justice noted that, to increase reporting, elder abuse has to be defined so that people know what it is. The provider needs to be aware of the definition, be aware of the laws regarding reporting, and have the knowledge and understanding of the next steps. Another workshop participant commented that the context in which the screening takes place is critical because if it is not done in a way that ensures trust and confidentiality, outcomes can be unpredictable, regardless of how good the tool is.

Although the EASI tool and much of the CMS work focus on screening in the primary care setting, workshop speaker Scott Beach from the University of Pittsburgh discussed screening for elder abuse in community-dwelling and institutional populations, drawing from work he and his colleagues have done as well as others. Table 5-1 lists different screening methods for community-dwelling and institutional populations, with members who are either cognitively intact or cognitively impaired.

Speaker Daniel Reingold from The Hebrew Home in Riverdale, New York, noted that facility staff have found screening is a very effective tool for elder abuse detection at the facility. The Hebrew Home has implemented mandatory elder abuse screening because so many victims come out of the hospital into postacute care without yet being detected. Through screening, they have identified more than 15 victims of elder abuse.

TABLE 5-1 Elder Abuse Screening and Detection: Overview

Community Dwelling: Cognitively Intact	Community Dwelling: Cognitively Impaired
• Direct victim surveys (random sample) • Direct victim surveys (targeted disease) • Direct caregiver surveys (targeted disease) • Direct perpetrator surveys (?) • Community "sentinels" (NEAIS) • Health care screening (physicians, emergency department, hospital, dental clinics) • Social service providers (adult day care) • Forensic analysis (bruising) • APS/official reports	• Direct caregiver surveys (targeted disease) • Direct perpetrator surveys (?) • Community "sentinels" (NEAIS) • Health care screening (physicians, ER, hospital, dental clinics) • Social service providers (adult day care) • Forensic analysis (bruising) • Adult Protective Services (APS)/official reports • Mild cognitive impairment—able to self-report?
Institutionalized/Long-Term Care (LTC): Cognitively Intact	Institutionalized/LTC: Cognitively Impaired
• Resident surveys • Family surveys • Resident informant/proxy surveys • Staff surveys • Video monitoring of public areas (?) • Forensic analysis (bruising) • LTC ombudsman/official reports (both staff–resident and resident–resident abuse)	• Family surveys • Resident informant/proxy surveys • Staff surveys • Video monitoring of public areas (?) • Forensic analysis (bruising) • LTC ombudsman/official reports (both staff–resident and resident–resident abuse)

NOTE: ER = emergency room; NEAIS = National Elder Abuse Incidence Study.
SOURCE: Beach, 2013.

Beach raised several issues and challenges he identified in conducting elder abuse screening:

- Who is being asked? Potential victims, clinicians, caregivers, proxies?
- Should the victim's perspective always be included when he or she is cognitively intact?
- What tool should be used?
- How should the data be collected: self-administered, through an interview, or through technology?
- Considering privacy and comfort, in what setting should it be administered?
- What method should be used to screen for neglect and self-neglect? Or financial exploitation?
- How should cultural context inform the screening?

Considering the breadth of existing tools, several workshop speakers stressed the use of learning and adapting from existing tools and their evidence rather than reinventing the wheel. Workshop speaker Ronald Acierno from the University of South Carolina noted, "We have basic building blocks. We have what has been demonstrated as a phenomenal way of detection. We have the setting where you have shown where you can do it, and people get together to combine those methods."

PREVENTION

Despite the magnitude of elder abuse around the world, little is known about how to prevent it before it occurs or how to stop it once it starts. Elder abuse is witnessed in many settings, and multiple sectors recognize the need to intervene. Some have started to take action; however, their efforts could be strengthened through increased knowledge sharing among stakeholders. Others are unsure of how to respond and need the tools to be able to take action. To facilitate discussions about opportunities for prevention, workshop participants engaged in breakout sessions on potential strategies and considerations for prevention in different settings: health care, the community, the legal system, and the financial sector. Breakout group leaders facilitated the sessions and individual participants provided comments from their perspective. Specific interventions suggested from within these different sectors were discussed throughout the workshop (see Boxes 5-1, 5-2, 5-3, and 5-4).

> **BOX 5-1**
> **Elder Investment Fraud and Financial**
> **Exploitation Prevention Program: Training Health**
> **Professionals on Financial Exploitation**
>
> Workshop participant Don Blandin from Investor Protection Trust (IPT) described an IPT program, the Elder Investment Fraud and Financial Exploitation Prevention Program (EIFFE Prevention Program). IPT's mission is to educate investors by providing information needed to make informed investment decisions. The EIFFE Prevention Program works to educate health professionals on how to identify abuse or potential abuse against their elder patients, and how to refer at-risk patients to State Securities Regulators or the local Adult Protective Services. These health professionals are educated through continuing medical education events, and materials for both clinicians and patients are available on the EIFFE Prevention Program website. This program was raised as an example of a program that could potentially be adapted to the legal sector.
>
> SOURCE: Investor Protection Trust, http://www.investorprotection.org/ipt-activities/?fa=eiffe-pp.

Health Care

Within the context of health care, workshop breakout group facilitator Elsie Yan from the University of Hong Kong suggested that special attention needs to be paid to case management and the transition of care, for example, from hospital to home. Within that context, the use of a team approach and integrated partnership among different disciplines might be reinforced. Furthermore, training in interventions should target staff at all levels, including clinical and nonclinical. It was suggested during the session that curricula for different health disciplines should incorporate gerontological approaches to case management and elder abuse training. It was also suggested that health providers should inform individuals of their choices, for example, of the use of and distinctions among advanced directives, guardianship, and their right of self-determination.

When considering opportunities for prevention in the community, health care providers such as dentists are well positioned to intervene. Recognizing that within institutional settings most violence occurs between residents, increasing staff–patient ratios and changing the environment were suggested as opportunities for prevention. Another recommendation from a breakout participant was to promote options for counseling to the caregivers and inform them of the continuum of care and quality of nursing home care to help them in decision making.

> **BOX 5-2**
> **Legal System Interventions**
>
> Lori Stiegel from the American Bar Association Commission on Law and Aging provided an overview of opportunities for the legal system to intervene and prevent elder abuse. These interventions exist at criminal, civil, and judicial levels and include
>
> - Criminal justice system at the local, state, and federal levels: Law enforcement, prosecutors, corrections, community corrections, victim services (both system and community based), and victim compensation;
> - Civil justice system: Public services lawyers (e.g., legal aid, law school clinics, and pro bono law) and private lawyers (e.g., elder law, probate and trust, and family law); and
> - Judicial system: State and federal courts.
>
> Participants in each of these systems have opportunities to prevent, detect, and remedy elder abuse. For example, civil lawyers can screen for elder abuse and counsel clients about how to prevent elder abuse. They can also prepare or revoke documents, such as powers of attorney, and can bring litigation in order to protect or recover a victim's assets. Civil lawyers need to become more educated about and involved in efforts to prevent and detect elder abuse. The criminal justice system can play a critical role in detecting and preventing elder abuse through policing, punishment, restitution to victims, and supervision of offenders.
>
> Judicial guidelines and standards, training, and tools for handling elder abuse cases have been developed by some organizations, such as the American Bar Association, the Florida International University, and the National Center for State Courts.
>
> Limited resources have been developed for and within each of these systems to help professionals learn how to recognize and handle elder abuse cases. There are sporadic trainings for participants in the three systems, but there is great need for more resources, particularly for civil lawyers.
>
> Special services are another way that law can intervene in elder abuse. For example, one criminal intervention is special prosecution units focusing on elder

Legal System

Workshop breakout facilitator Charles Sabatino from the American Bar Association commented that the legal system traditionally becomes involved later in cases of elder abuse rather than in primary prevention. The focus in primary prevention has been heavily on education and training and the competencies needed to screen for and detect abuse and exploitation as well as addressing it early and in many cases divert it from the legal system. He suggested that the stakeholders who should be targeted for training in abuse. Some areas of the country have well-known units, such as Brooklyn, Manhattan, San Diego, and Seattle; in most of the United States, however, it is rare to find someone in a prosecutor's office who knows about and understands elder abuse, and even more rare to find a specialized unit. Within the judicial system, court-focused elder abuse initiatives are a recent development. Examples of such initiatives include elder protection courts (special dockets for elder abuse cases) and elder protection order projects that enable older homebound persons to petition for protection orders by telephone.

Elder abuse multidisciplinary teams, such as elder abuse forensic centers, provide another opportunity for criminal and civil lawyers to prevent elder abuse and to improve systems. A recent study demonstrates that cases reviewed by elder abuse forensic centers have a 10 times greater likelihood of being presented to the district attorney (Navarro et al., 2013). However, because the criminal justice system is not focused on the needs of victims, it is important to include civil lawyers on multidisciplinary teams to ensure consideration of civil legal tools that may benefit victims. There is great opportunity for future research on the intervention of multidisciplinary teams.

The corrections and community corrections systems provide additional opportunities for prevention and intervention. It can be expensive to care for elderly prisoners, and a recent trend is to release old and ill prisoners. The possibility of elder abuse and family violence should be considered in this policy issue. A similar issue arises in the community corrections system, where professionals have an opportunity to direct offenders coming out of prison away from working in nursing homes or assisted living facilities, and to assess whether additional supervision might be warranted if an offender is living with elderly parents or grandparents.

Finally, it is important for the public and the professionals who serve them to be aware that—contrary to what they see on television—in the criminal justice system a crime is actually committed against the state, and victims are considered to be witnesses to that crime; it is up to the state to determine whether an alleged perpetrator of elder abuse should be prosecuted.

For more information, see http://www.elderabuseforensiccenter.com.

SOURCE: Lori Stiegel, American Bar Association Commission on Law and Aging.

---

legal interventions and opportunities for prevention are police, prosecutors, judges, and other professionals that are connected to the legal system, such as those in protective services and at financial institutions. The legal system and the courts often are part of an insular culture and are not naturally inclined to go out of their comfort zone; however, elder abuse prevention involves many sectors and collaboration is suggested to increase the effectiveness of prevention efforts.

A second issue that Sabatino reported on was guardianship. Guardianship often is seen in legal theory as a remedy for abuse and neglect and for

> **BOX 5-3**
> **The Hebrew Home at Riverdale:**
> **A Community-Based Intervention**
>
> Workshop speaker Daniel Reingold from The Hebrew Home at Riverdale in New York presented the elder abuse shelter model that was developed at The Hebrew Home and has been replicated in other locations. He emphasized that the community is required to create an elder abuse shelter; it is a collaborative model that uses the existing resources of a community. In particular, using a nonprofit long-term care facility, a nursing home is one of the greatest models and one of the reasons that internally within a long-term care facility there is an existing community that can be used to shelter, protect, and empower victims of elder abuse. The model is nimble and flexible and can be adapted to the specific community. (See *Reingold et al.* in Part II of this report for an in-depth discussion of the elder abuse shelter model.)
>
> SOURCE: Daniel Reingold, The Hebrew Home at Riverdale.

issues of inadequate capacity, but it is often a part of the problem rather than the solution. It is frequently overused and courts tend to see guardianship as a black-and-white choice. Sabatino suggested that other intervention resources within the legal system could be more important, but are generally underfunded. There is often a lack of structure for various legal tools that could prevent elder abuse in the first place, particularly around powers of attorney and legal tools. Frequently this is the result of weak state laws or a lack of lawyer training in elder abuse, for example, when counseling clients on estate planning. Expanded use of ombudsman planning is another adjunct resource that could be helpful. Along with these resources and the courts, the lack of knowing what happens in these cases is a chronic problem. There are poor data systems and they tend to focus on the front and on how many cases were filed; often it is unknown what happens to these cases after they enter the system. One suggestion that came from a breakout group participant was mandating minimum institutional staffing ratios.

Community-Based

Breakout session facilitator Joy Solomon from The Hebrew Home at Riverdale provided some reflections from the community-based breakout discussions. She suggested that the most important question that was raised during the discussion was "What is community?" How community is defined affects prevention efforts and where in the community they occur. She noted that several breakout session participants suggested there may be valuable lessons learned in the area of community-based prevention

> **BOX 5-4**
> **OWN IT: Wells Fargo Advisors and**
> **Financial Exploitation Prevention**
>
> Ronald Long from Wells Fargo Advisors (WFA) presented WFA's efforts to prevent elder financial exploitation. Recognizing that elders are targets for financial exploitation, WFA has put significant resources toward building its capacity to prevent it. WFA's efforts include training most of its employees, a centralized response unit, client-focused information, educational outreach, and partnerships. They have developed the **OWN IT** model to raise awareness among their employees and empower them to act when they detect exploitation:
>
> - **Observe:** Are there physical changes? Are patterns and habits different? How is the elder around the third-party person present?
> - **Wonder Why:** Why are withdrawal multiples larger than before? Why is money sent to a new country?
> - **Negotiate:** Can the transaction go later? Can the check go in two names, elder and trusted third party? Can we only give a fraction of the money today and more later?
> - **Isolate:** Get the elder alone: "Ms. Smith, please step with me to confirm some account information" or "Please come with me to discuss some confidential information."
> - **Tattle:** Bring concerns to manager immediately. Use firm's Adult Protective Services reporting process.
>
> (See *Long* in Part II of this report for an in depth discussion of WFA's model.)
>
> SOURCE: Ronald Long, Wells Fargo Advisors.

from the fields of domestic violence and child abuse. Solomon reflected that the value of coalitions and the role of multidisciplinary teams is an important theme that has come up throughout the workshop. She stressed that within the community context, where there are many actors, multidisciplinary work is extremely important across different agencies but even within one agency. Workshop planning committee member and breakout session co-facilitator Jeffrey Hall from the Centers for Disease Control and Prevention observed from the breakout discussion that people use different jargon. In the context of community-based interventions, particularly ones that involve multidisciplinary teams, understanding different definitions of "community" is important for developing partnerships. He added that a key factor for moving forward will be the use of non-traditional partnerships to bring groups and individuals to the table in ways they have not in the past. At the same time that different stakeholder groups are being embraced, older adults themselves should be taught about prevention.

Solomon noted that there can be tension in the area of community-based intervention implementation between the "just do it" model and waiting for the evidence model. Hall suggested that, while the movement to build the evidence base for elder abuse and its prevention is underway, action will be needed. A reasonable accommodation would be to have guided exploration of particular interventions to address elder abuse and allow the collection of information to compile the evidence base for which future interventions can be launched. Commenting on the idea of frameworks, Hall cautioned that it is important to not allow frameworks to become barriers. The conversations about elder abuse prevention need to include multiple perspectives and use inclusive concepts.

Financial Sector

Workshop participant Naomi Karp from the Consumer Financial Protection Bureau provided some comments based on her participation in the financial sector breakout session. She noted that several of the session participants discussed the challenges of information sharing in financial exploitation prevention efforts. For example, when the front-line financial sector professionals detect what they suspect may be elder financial exploitation, they often have concerns about what information they can share with government entities and others without violating privacy rules. She said a number of federal agencies are making an effort to provide some clarification and guidance on information sharing and privacy protection. Karp also noted that there was discussion about enhancing the use of suspicious activity reports (SARs) at financial institutions. Now that there is a category for elder financial exploitation, efforts should be made to better collection data and share information based on the SARs.

Karp mentioned the need for financial institutions to delay transactions or freeze accounts when there is suspected abuse, and said it would be helpful if there was a catalogue of state remedies already in place. Karp also noted that financial institutions often have concerns about reporting and being held liable; state laws on mandatory reporting and related immunity provisions need to be made known. She also noted the Financial Services Roundtable has a new training curriculum for financial institutions that can provide vital information.

REFERENCES

Beach, S. 2013. *Screening and detection.* Presented at Elder Abuse and Its Prevention: A Workshop. Institute of Medicine, Washington, DC, April 18.

Navarro, A. E., Z. D. Gassoumis, and K. H. Wilber. 2013. Holding abusers accountable: An elder abuse forensic center increases criminal prosecution of financial exploitation. *Gerontologist* 53(2):303-312.

6

The Way Forward

To move the field of elder abuse research and prevention forward, innovative ideas are needed that will contribute to the evidence base, raise awareness, change attitudes, and provide the necessary tools to take action. At the close of the workshop, several speakers provided comments on the progress of health policy and awareness building toward these ends. Additionally, several speakers provided their reflections based on the discussions over the course of the 2 days on priority areas for moving the field forward. This chapter includes summaries of the comments they provided.

HEALTH POLICY AND PROMOTING AWARENESS

Workshop planning committee member and moderator Edwin Walker from the Administration on Aging acknowledged that elder abuse is no longer an invisible problem. Solutions can be developed collectively that bring about the cultural change necessary to globally address the issue and build systems that are truly responsive. Workshop speakers discussed elder abuse prevention through international collaboration, policy-level efforts in the United States, and increased awareness.

The International Network for the Prevention of Elder Abuse

Susan Somers from the International Network for the Prevention of Elder Abuse (INPEA) presented on INPEA's global efforts. INPEA, which includes representation from 60 countries, aims to increase the ability of societies to recognize and respond to mistreatment of older persons across settings through international collaboration. Considering the diversity of the cultures represented within their membership, reflecting on cultural relevance is an important aspect of their work. INPEA's objectives are to

- promote education and training of professionals and paraprofessionals in identification, treatment, and prevention;
- further advocacy on behalf of abused and neglected elders; and
- stimulate research into the causes, consequences, prevalence, treatment, and prevention of elder abuse and neglect.

Collaboration with the United Nations

INPEA has nongovernmental organization (NGO) special consultative status to the United Nations (UN) Economic and Social Council and is given 2 or 3 minutes at every other session to speak. In 2008, INPEA organized a program on social isolation, which was the first time this issue was discussed at the UN. INPEA also has participated in the 2002 UN Second World Assembly on Ageing in Madrid, the Intergovernmental Conferences on Ageing for the 5-year regional follow-ups to Madrid, and the International Plan of Action on Ageing. The organization's key UN strategies and challenges include

- building knowledge and capacity of NGOs and Member States and Older Persons;
- maximizing awareness of consequences of ageism, inequality, and gender discrimination;
- seeking out and sharing effective, evidence-based sustainable solutions; and
- identifying key stakeholders for collaboration.

World Elder Abuse Awareness Day

The World Elder Abuse Awareness Day (WEAAD) was first instituted by INPEA on June 15, 2006. On December 19, 2011, the UN General Assembly officially recognized elder abuse as a global social issue that affects the health and human rights of millions of older persons around the world.

Urgent Concerns

Somers noted several urgent concerns in the area of elder abuse globally that INPEA has identified as priorities moving forward:

- violence against older women/widows;
- harmful cultural and traditional practices;
- lack of social protection;
- extreme poverty;
- self-neglect; and
- dementia.

The Elder Justice Act and Policy-Level Efforts in the United States

Robert Blancato from the Elder Justice Coalition presented on progress toward elder justice through policy efforts in the United States. The Elder Justice Act (EJA) was introduced in 2002 and 2003 and had grown out of hearings and the related work of the Senate Special Committee on Aging. The bill was motivated by two factors: (1) less than 2 percent of federal funds for violence prevention were being spent on elder abuse; and (2) no single person in the entire federal government worked on elder abuse. The EJA was the subject of numerous hearings in the Senate and House and passed in the Senate Finance Committee on three different occasions. Finally, in 2010, it became law as an amendment to the Patient Protection and Affordable Care Act (see Box 6-1 for details on the law). Since its passage, work has begun to secure funding for the authorizations in the bill; implement the law, and work to pass parts of the original bill that were not included, such as the Elder Abuse Victims Act.

Blancato noted that 2012 was a year of progress. That year the White House held a high-level WEAAD event; new grants were awarded to test best practices going forward, including funding to tribal organizations; and

---

BOX 6-1
Features of the Elder Justice Act

- Authorization of $777 million over 4 years in the areas of Adult Protective Services (APS) funding, state demonstration grants, long-term care ombudsman program, long-term care staffing support, training programs, improved data collection and dissemination, and research related to APS;
- Establishment of the Elder Justice Coordinating Council, which makes recommendations to the Secretary of the Department of Health and Human Services on the coordination of activities of federal, state, local, and private agencies and entities relating to elder abuse, neglect, and exploitation; and
- Establishment of a 27-member Advisory Board on Elder Abuse, Neglect and Exploitation, which has yet to be named or convened.

the Elder Justice Coordinating Council was convened, providing an opportunity for governmental agencies to share with each other the work they are doing. In addition, in 2012, the President's budget included EJA funding for the second year in a row and the Department of Justice continued to work on the roadmap project. Blancato suggested that the range of related bills introduced in 2012 shows interest on a bipartisan basis (see Box 6-2).

Blancato noted progress that has continued in 2013:

- Violence Against Women Reauthorization Act of 2013 passed with elder abuse funding.
- Elder Abuse Victims Act of 2013 was introduced.
- First elder abuse hearing of this Congress's Senate Aging Committee was held on March 13; the second was held on April 10.
- Senate Budget Resolution passed with Amendment No. 594 supporting the Older Americans Act, including Title VII.

While progress is being made, Blancato also illuminated several areas where work still needs to be done: funding the EJA; implementing the rest of the EJA (including the Elder Justice Advisory Council, the designated home for Adult Protective Services in the Department of Health and Human Services, data collection, enforcement of Centers for Medicare & Medicaid Services guidelines on reporting crimes in nursing homes, and more state applications for grants for criminal background checks); reintroducing 2012 bills in the 113th Congress and getting new movement; and passing the Older Americans Act.

BOX 6-2
Elder Justice-Related Bills Introduced in the 112th Congress

- Elder Abuse Victims Act (S. 462) (Sen. Kohl)
- Senior Financial Empowerment Act (S. 465) (Sen. Gillibrand)
- National Silver Alert Act (H.R. 112, S. 1263) (Rep. Doggett, Sen. Kohl)
- Elder Protection and Abuse Prevention Act (S. 2077) (Sen. Blumenthal)
- Older Americans Act Reauthorization 2012 (S. 3562) (second attempt in 2012) (Sen. Sanders)
- LGBT Elder Americans Act of 2012 (S. 3575), amendment to Older Americans Act (Sen. Bennet)
- Robert Matava Exploitation Protection for Elder Adults Act of 2012 (S. 3598) (Sen. Blumenthal)
- Improving Dementia Care Treatment in Older Adults Act (S. 3604) (Sen. Kohl)

Blancato provided several comments about the effects of sequestration on elder abuse prevention efforts. Sequestration cuts are affecting elder abuse detection programs around the country, including the Social Services Block Grant, which supports APS. Additionally, cuts to Title VII programs are in the double digits in some states. Blancato noted that sequestration could end starting in fiscal year 2014; however, in the worst case scenario, it could continue for another 9 years.

Reflecting on progress made to date, Blancato suggested that it has been possible due to leadership in the President's Administration and bipartisan leadership in Congress, as well as sustained national state and local advocacy. The Elder Justice Coalition was founded 10 years ago and served to coordinate advocacy at the national level. It had 5 founding organizations and has grown to 3,000 members. Furthermore, media coverage has aided in the effort, especially of celebrated cases such as Brooke Astor and Mickey Rooney.

Going forward, particularly in a time of sequestration and deficit reduction, advocacy must be more aggressive, stressing prevention, and state of the art. The Elder Justice Coalition is starting a collaboration with the Ageless Alliance to increase visibility of elder justice through social media.

To make progress toward prevention, investments should be made in programs that target prevention and also save funding in other federal programs such as Medicaid and Medicare. Furthermore, because what is not reported cannot be stopped, investments need to be made in better detection, more reporting, and more resources to the entities where elder abuse is reported.

Elder abuse also needs to be recognized as a growing women's issue, as well as a baby boomers' issue. The average victim is an older woman living alone; nearly half of all women over 75 live alone. Baby boomers control 70 percent of disposable income in the United States and first-wave boomers are now 67.

Blancato noted that the Elder Justice Act expires in 2014, so 2013 is a pivotal year to show its value. Despite the progress that has been made to date, there is still much progress to be done. Going forward, the work that has been started by Congress and the Obama Administration needs to continue to push the field of elder abuse prevention forward.

Enhancing the Public Health Response: Priority Policy Issues

Marie-Therese Connolly,
Woodrow Wilson International Center for Scholars

Workshop speaker Marie-Therese Connolly reflected back to the 2007 Institute of Medicine (IOM) workshop on Preventing Violence in Low- and

Middle-Income Countries, which was the founding event in the IOM beginning work to address violence prevention through the Forum on Global Violence Prevention. She remarked that at that workshop, elder abuse was an afterthought. While the field still has a long way to go, the workshop on elder abuse and its prevention in 2013 shows that it is no longer an afterthought. To continue to move the field of elder abuse forward, Connelly suggested seven actions, which are listed below and described in detail in *Connolly and Trilling* in Part II of this report:

1. develop policy to recognize elder abuse as a public health issue;
2. address research priorities critical to inform policy and practice: intervention, defining success, prevention, data collection, and cost;
3. translate what we know into practice;
4. address the resources issue;
5. implement law and developing policy infrastructure;
6. develop a political constituency; and
7. promote innovation.

MOVING PREVENTION FORWARD

Based on the discussions they observed and participated in during the 2-day workshop, several speakers provided comments from their perspective on priority issues for moving the field of elder abuse prevention forward.

Reflections from a U.S. Government Perspective
U.S. Assistant Secretary of Aging Kathy Greenlee, Administration on Aging

As a member of the Forum on Global Violence Prevention since its founding in 2010, Administration on Aging Assistant Secretary Kathy Greenlee expressed her appreciation to the IOM and her Forum colleagues for undertaking a workshop on elder abuse and its prevention. While elder abuse has been part of the Forum's work through its activities, dedicating a full workshop to it has shed light on a type of violence that often takes a backseat to other more readily recognized forms of violence, such as child abuse and intimate partner violence. Greenlee also expressed her appreciation to her colleagues from other U.S. government agencies who attended and participated in the event, demonstrating the multisectoral dedication to elder abuse prevention.

Conceptual Framework

Greenlee noted that Pamela Teaster's presentation on conceptual frameworks was helpful and showed that there is no structure by which work in this field is being analyzed. As the development of a conceptual framework moves forward, Greenlee offered two thoughts to consider. She suggested that part of the success in the work of domestic violence has been the critical support and training it took to include law enforcement. Elder abuse is a crime and whatever theoretical framework is developed, it has to be something that can translate to law enforcement, prosecutors, and judges so that the framework supports the understanding of elder abuse as a criminal activity. The other thought she offered about the framework was on the public health model. Greenlee noted that as a lawyer by training and public servant, she has struggled with applying the public health structure and the categorization of primary, secondary, and tertiary prevention to elder abuse because of ageism. Articulating primary prevention for older people can be very hard to do; some people incorrectly assume by the time someone has reached old age, primary prevention is too late or not feasible. She posited putting the model on its head with tertiary first and then secondary and then primary because primary is such a struggle. Greenlee suggested that if a framework can be developed that achieves these objectives of being inclusive of law enforcement and creating a practical public health approach, she could work with any structure that is developed.

Inclusion of Individuals with Disabilities

Greenlee noted that in addition to serving as Assistant Secretary for Aging, she also serves as Administrator for the Administration on Community Living (ACL). ACL serves people with disabilities and older adults as well as their families through what she refers to as a multicultural approach to aging and disability. She suggested that as work in the area of elder abuse moves forward, it needs to be done in a way that addresses the needs of people with disabilities who are not older and actually includes people with disabilities themselves. Alzheimer's disease affects people of all ages even though there is a higher prevalence of people who are older, as does Parkinson's disease and multiple sclerosis. Greenlee asked: "How can we make sure that when we tackle the twin pillars of cognitive impairment and social isolation, it is inclusive of people with disabilities?"

Elder Justice Act and Adult Protective Services

The fact that the Elder Justice Act has not been funded is a tremendous problem on which Greenlee will continue to work. Blancato mentioned the desire for a designated federal home for Adult Protective Services, and Greenlee suggested that it could be possible to fund it through the Older Americans Act because elder abuse has always been incorporated into the goals of the Older Americans Act. However, she noted the limitations of funding and the amount of resources she can put toward it without Elder Justice Act funding.

The Twin Pillars

Greenlee also noted that while much can be learned from other fields, such as mental health, domestic violence, and child abuse, two issues must be addressed specifically in the area of elder abuse—cognitive impairment and social isolation.

Based on the content of the presentations and discussions throughout the workshop, Greenlee suggested that, in fact, there are assets at hand to work on moving elder abuse prevention forward. Although the field has "more brains than money," she is optimistic that it will move forward.

Reflections from a Research Perspective

Terry Fulmer, Northeastern University

Be Proactive in Building the Evidence

Speaker and planning committee member Dr. Terry Fulmer suggested that, despite the fact that researchers in the field are highly critical of the research progress to date, the evidence base is moving forward. To continue the progress, she suggested that researchers should define the key elder abuse constructs and variables that we need to examine instead of waiting for others, such as policy makers or legal systems to define them, and establish the metrics and data to move ahead. Investigators should share their data and allow others to critique those data in order to strengthen the national and international science of elder mistreatment. Variability in approaches to data collection and nomenclature need to be examined, but also appreciated as there are multiple "ways of knowing." Fulmer further noted that there is a clear imperative to move the Elder Justice Act and its reauthorization forward. She further recognized that approaches to research on elder mistreatment are challenging and more national and international collaborations need to take place to move the science forward.

Create Partnerships

Fulmer suggested that where collective partnerships are missing, they should be created. Stronger research relationships with the adult protective service system are urgently needed and strategies must be created to protect the privacy of individuals while using the data available through APS and other data systems such as electronic health records to study the problem and make progress in interventions that can work. Research in the field of elder abuse and elder abuse prevention is all-consuming and researchers need to be able to reach out to their colleagues for support and encouragement. In terms of developing work groups and research teams in areas such as measurement, Fulmer commented that rather than solely waiting for conference grants or other sources of funding, investigators need to push forward and start sharing by connecting through conference calls, Web-based video calls, and other lower cost strategies.

Take Programs Where They Are

Fulmer commented that throughout the workshop, promising intervention programs were presented: some are just starting and others are accelerating. She suggested that these intervention programs, such as the work that is being done at the Harry and Jeanette Weinberg Center for Elder Abuse Prevention at The Hebrew Home at Riverdale, need to be replicated, further researched, and continuously improved.

Fulmer also noted that, in the field of elder abuse, we have a great deal of evidence that is known and it should be used. She asked the participants to take not only what they have learned collectively during the workshop, but what they know from their disciplines, practices, and programs of research and move the evidence forward. She finally underscored the global nature of the workshop discussions, the inclusion of new and multiple perspectives, and expressed enthusiasm and optimism for future global collaborations.

Reflections from a Global Perspective
Greg Shaw, International Federation of Ageing

Workshop speaker Greg Shaw noted that, although elder abuse research is happening all over the world, the challenge that he often grapples with is, "How do we capture it and make networks much more effective across the world? What new suspicion index is being developed? Where can we build from the best of the best? . . . Where do we get a repository or clearinghouse with some interaction around discussion forums where groups can come together to start talking about what they are doing in the field?" He suggested that these are important challenges to address, because the more knowledge is shared, the more power there will be to effect change. Several other challenges in moving elder abuse prevention forward that Shaw mentioned were making it a public health priority, educating health professionals, focusing on community-level efforts, and involving youth.

Public Health Priority

Shaw suggested the need to make elder abuse a priority public health problem that is recognized along with noncommunicable diseases as an area where resources should be devoted in the future.

Education and Training for Health Professionals

Health professionals are confronted all the time by cases of elder abuse, yet often they fail to recognize them. When they do, they often do not know where to go or how to handle the problem. Shaw suggested more research on screening tools and training for health professionals.

Community-Level Efforts

Several innovative community-level efforts were discussed during the workshop, such as the virtual shelter model and a training program for door attendants in Brazil. Shaw asked: "How can we build on creative community-level models? How do we interact with the people who know what is happening in their own communities, whether it's hairdressers, door [attendants], or other community members?"

Involving Youth

Shaw suggested that if a movement among youth can be fostered around identifying and understanding what elder abuse is, perhaps in the future, elder abuse can be prevented before it starts.

Part II

Papers and Commentary from Speakers

II.1

UNDERSTANDING ELDER ABUSE IN THE CHINESE COMMUNITY: THE ROLE OF CULTURAL, SOCIAL, AND COMMUNITY FACTORS

E-Shien Chang, M.A., XinQi Dong, M.D., M.P.H.
Chinese Health, Aging, and Policy Program,
Rush Institute for Healthy Aging
Rush University Medical Center

Introduction

With an estimated population of 1.3 billion people, China has the largest population in the world. Since its reform in 1978, China has experienced rapid economic growth and an increase in life expectancy, while the population as a whole is aging. Chinese older adults account for the world's largest aging population with 143 million people aged 60 years and older (Leng et al., 2008). By 2050, approximately one-third of China's population will be over age 60, accounting for one-quarter of the world's aging population. In the United States, the Chinese American community is the oldest, largest, and among the fastest growing Asian subpopulation (Bennett and Martin, 1995; Barnes and Bennett, 2002). From 2000 to 2010, the Chinese elderly population aged 65 and over has experienced a growth rate nearly four times higher than America's older population (U.S. Census Bureau, 2011).

The dramatic growth of the global Chinese aging population has important implications for the health care, social welfare, justice, and financial systems. With this trend comes the potential for greater increased rates of elder abuse. However, the issue of cultural diversity surrounding elder abuse is an increasing challenge to this field of research. Despite ongoing efforts of multiple disciplines across academic, community, state, and federal organizations, we have a limited understanding of cultural and social issues of elder abuse in Chinese populations worldwide. We need to better examine the cultural variations in the construct, definition, and perception of elder abuse (Moon and Williams, 1993; Moon et al., 2002). In addition, there are knowledge gaps in in-depth cultural explorations of the barriers to elder abuse interventions and help-seeking behaviors with respect to the specific social and cultural contexts (Dong et al., 2007b).

Cultural Traditions: Filial Piety

Chinese traditional culture has been heavily influenced by Confucian traditions, which greatly emphasize filial piety, and these ethical principles provide guidelines regarding power, roles, and responsibilities of each family member. In the teachings of Confucius, filial piety (孝 Xiào) dictates children's obligatory roles and responsibilities of caregiving to aging parents. As a well-known Chinese proverb states, "Raising children is protective against older age and frailty" (養兒防老 Yǎng-Er-Fáng-Lǎo) (Lan, 2002; Mencius and Lau, 2005). In return, parents are expected to contribute to the harmony of family and society with their guidance and wisdom.

For thousands of years, this system of interdependence among family members has worked well for Chinese society. However, the processes of modernization, urbanization, and industrialization have generated greater mobility of adult children from rural to urban settings in China, which in turn have altered changes in family structures and expected intergenerational filial support of older adults. There is evidence, however, that the younger generations of Chinese are less adherent to traditional Confucian principles of filial piety (Tsai, 1999; Ng et al., 2002). As a result, elderly Chinese are no longer guaranteed prestige, power, and care in the family, and they may be forced into stressful adjustments in their lives. The tradition of filial piety has been now made and monitored by the Chinese government as a legal contract, in which violations will be subjected to penalties by law (Chou, 2010).

In the context of immigration, whereas many Chinese American families are transforming from traditional Chinese collective culture to Western society's emphasis on individualism (Mui, 1996; Casado and Leung, 2001), acculturation stress, access to health care, and linguistic and cultural barriers may pose great challenges to the families and their traditional values (Casado and Leung, 2001; Tam and Neysmith, 2006). Research suggests that the cultural ideal of filial piety is continually practiced with varying provisions, depending on local circumstances of historical, social, and familial configurations (Ikels, 2004). However, these transformations may threaten the support system of Chinese older adults, which can further exacerbate vulnerability, physical dependency, and psychological distress, and reflect conditions that strongly contribute to the increased risk for elder abuse.

Cultural and Linguistic Diversity

A major complexity in advancing the field of elder abuse among the Chinese population is exemplified by the issues of cultural and linguistic diversity. As the most populous country in the world, China is also inherently diverse. Although the majority Han group constitutes 91 percent of the total population, China's other 55 minority nationalities amount to 123.3 million people, which is roughly equivalent to 40 percent of the U.S. population (U.S. Census Bureau, 2009). Linguistic diversity as a by-product was well developed (Xu and Wang, 2007). These forms of speech, according to a renowned Chinese linguist, could be as far apart as English to Dutch, or French to Italian (Chao, 1976). In the case of the U.S. Chinese population, less than one-third of the Chinese American community was born in the United States; nearly half of Chinese Americans speak English less than very well (Shinagawa, 2008). Not only are the language and cultural barriers challenging, Chinese communities are diverse due to the history and development of immigration trajectories (Moreno-John et al., 2004; Parikh et al., 2009). These sociodemographic characteristics further call for culturally sensitive measures for researchers in the field of elder abuse (Norman, 1988; Wong, 1998; Guo, 2000; Shinagawa, 2008).

Prevalence of Elder Abuse

Prior studies in the People's Republic of China suggest that abuse of older persons is common (Yan and Tang, 2001; Dong et al., 2007b). Caregiver neglect was the most common form of abuse, followed by financial exploitation, psychological abuse, physical abuse, sexual abuse, and abandonment. Of the victims in the study sample, 36 percent suffered from multiple forms of abuse and neglect (Dong et al., 2007b). In a large population-based study of 3,018 Chinese community-dwelling adults aged 60 and older in the greater Chicago area, 24 percent experienced elder abuse since they turned 60. Despite its common existence, elder abuse remains underrecognized among Chinese older adults due to high cultural sensitivity, low level of awareness, reluctance to reveal the case to maintain family harmony and honor, and the perception that elder abuse is a private family matter (Yan and Tang, 2001; Dong et al., 2007b).

Cultural Perceptions of Elder Abuse

Evidence suggests that older adults from different racial/ethnic groups have varying levels of tolerance toward different types of abuse (National Center on Elder Abuse, 1999). Moreover, there has been little qualitative information to provide deeper understanding of the threshold and tolerability of abuse in different racial/ethnic groups. In the first community-based participatory research (CBPR) study of elder abuse among Chinese older adults in Chicago, elder abuse was frequently characterized in terms of caregiver neglect (Dong et al., 2011b). As an older adult described, "Older adults are too frail to work outside. They don't speak the language (English). They depend on their children for help. If the children do not help, then the older adults will have no one to turn to." Financial exploitation, physical abuse, and abandonment were considered serious as well. However, psychological abuse, including verbal and emotional abuse, was perceived to be more serious than other forms of abuse. As a study participant reported, "the most serious one is psychological abuse, like saying, go to die early. Cursing is abusive because it makes people sad." This is to say, although Chinese older adults were aware of the brutality of physical abuse, they placed more concern toward psychological mistreatment, which fundamentally violates the filial obligations under the influence of Confucius's teachings. Hence, Chinese older adults may hold higher emotional expectations for their adult children, and may be more prone to emotional distress when the expectation is unmet. The emphasis on caregiver neglect and psychological abuse may be affected by the belief in traditional familial obligations.

Perceived Psychosocial Impact of Elder Abuse

Research suggests that the discrepancies between expectations and actual receipts of care may be detrimental to Chinese older adults' psychological and social well-being and is further associated with elder abuse. A number of exploratory studies reported the perceived psychosocial impact of elder abuse from the perspectives of Chinese older adults (Dong et al., 2012a,b). Based on the findings of a qualitative study with community-dwelling older adults in Chicago, depressive symptoms were associated with adverse health consequences from physical, cognitive, and mental health perspectives (Dong et al., 2012a). Its results suggest that older adults with depressive symptoms were more likely to associate depression with suicidal thoughts and elder abuse than those who did not report any symptoms. As an older adult reported, "My thought is that depressed seniors may sit at home and feel helpless. What if then they are ill treated by their children? That would make the situation even more alarming." Moreover, loneliness and worsening social isolation have been reported as adverse health outcomes of abuse in the Chinese population (Dong et al., 2012b). In particular, elder abuse may be a major contributing factor in the feeling of loneliness, while conversely, loneliness may also increase the risk of being abused by a trusted other (Dong and Simon, 2007b).

More importantly, from the viewpoints of Chinese older adults, elder abuse was associated with increases in suicidal ideation and behaviors (Dong et al., 2012a). The sense of shame and cultural stigma on elder abuse may overshadow the motivations to seek interventions. When higher expectation was placed on family harmony, any violation would be deemed as a shame to the family. As a study participant described, "you might not agree with me. But sometimes when I feel bad about things I would rather swallow a pill and die as long as it is not too painful." In the United States, Chinese older adults were reported to have the highest suicide rate than any other ethnic groups nationwide. Specifically, the suicide rate among older Chinese women is a higher leading cause of death compared with the general population (Foo, 2003; CDC, 2010a,b). A prior study noted a three-fold higher suicide rate among Chinese women ages 65-74, seven-fold higher among those ages 75-84, and 10-fold higher among those over age 85 compared to white women of the same age groups (Liu and Yu, 1985; Yu et al., 1985).

Help-Seeking Tendency of Elder Abuse

Qualitative studies suggest that Chinese older adults commonly believed that abuse cases "had no solution"; others proposed "sending the victim away" (from the perpetrator); and still others stated that the fear of "losing face" would deter the reporting of elder abuse (Dong et al., 2011a). The violation of a trusting relationship between older adults and their family members was regarded as unsettling. As a study participant described, "How can we help this person? You may talk about it only with your very close friends. Yet most people would neither talk about it nor report it. They would only blame their own children and cry."

However, the dominance of stigma and fears as a barrier to seeking abuse intervention warrants more attention. Although this was attributable to the traditional Chinese cultural doctrine in family honors and pride, it may also be a consequence of the lack of culturally appropriate intervention programs (Sue et al., 2009). Culturally sensitive approaches to address these barriers will be critical to encourage victims to seek interventions. An initial strategy would involve programs specifically designed to reduce stigma associated with elder abuse and elder abuse interventions. Second, an approach to provide culturally adapted materials to increase older adults' awareness in elder abuse will be crucial. There is also a need to increase accessibility and availability of elder abuse interventions at a systematic level.

Community Support in Nurturing Filial Piety Values and Intergenerational Relationships

Studies on elder abuse help-seeking behaviors among Chinese older adults concurred that if elder abuse cases happened in the community, seeking assistance from community service organizations would be the most viable solution (Dong et al., 2011a). Because of the bilingual and bicultural social services that community organizations provide, study participants believed that "other than community service organizations, there is no other way to handle the cases." The indirect family-centered, community-based intervention preference among Chinese older adults is consistent with previous research in a Native American community where familism was also practiced (Holkup et al., 2007).

Specifically, future interventions would need to be directed toward enhancing social support of Chinese older adults, particularly in the form of family support. Social service agencies working with Chinese older adults should pay special notice to their social connectedness to adult children, intergenerational exchange, cultural expectations, and satisfaction with family. Community organizations with bilingual services and staff may play a pivotal role. On the one hand, social workers may help Chinese older adults establish an improved social network, better supporting relationships, and physical and mental health, thus reducing the risks of abuse. On the other hand, such organizations could help improve the capacity of family members to offer adequate care and prevent older adults from being isolated. Building a stronger association with people in their own community will provide emotional, social, and practical supports for the older immigrants. Consideration of these variables could be important to the design of culturally appropriate elder abuse interventions.

Community-Based Participatory Research Methodology

Taking culture into account is the prerequisite of delivering high-quality health care services to people from diverse sociocultural contexts (Kleinman et al., 1978; Tervalon, 2003). However, language and cultural barriers often complicate the ability of minority immigrants to understand and participate in research studies (Cristancho et al., 2008; Martinez et al., 2009). Concerning the highly sensitive nature of elder abuse issues among Chinese older adults, the ability to reach out to the community and investigate this health issue was facilitated using the CBPR approach. CBPR is particularly useful to studying the well-being of the minority population, whose health beliefs and behaviors are highly intertwined with their unique cultural insights (Israel, 2000; Minkler and Wallerstein, 2003; Minkler, 2005). By equally engaging both academic and community partners in an action-driven investigation, the quality and quantity of research is enhanced without losing sight of local community values.

Recent elder abuse research in Chinese communities has demonstrated success and has enhanced infrastructure and networks necessary for community-engaged research and community–academic collaborations (Dong et al., 2011a,c). Conducting the CBPR approach allows researchers to gain cultural awareness of community health and to develop appropriate prevention and intervention measures on elder abuse issues. Working with the Chinese community highlights the importance of respecting and embracing diverse cultural philosophies, practices, and preferences in sustaining partnerships. Genuine understanding and practice of culturally sensitive research are critical for advancing social change.

Meeting the Challenge of Cultural Complexity

Finally, it is imperative to vertically integrate cultural sensitivity training into the current health care professional training and education. Such curriculums should encourage health professionals to become better listeners and humble students of the older adults, which are essential steps to comprehend the cultural variations of health, aging, and elder abuse issues (Chang et al., 2010). Culturally appropriate training and resources for the Adult Protective Services (APS) and other front-line workers will also be critical to alleviate factors exacerbating abusive situations in the Chinese communities, and to prevent elder abuse recidivism.

Conclusion

Elder abuse is a pervasive public health issue, yet there are major gaps in understanding the cultural and social complexities with respect to elder abuse among the diverse Chinese population worldwide. We need representative longitudinal research to better define the incidence, risk/protective factors, and consequences of elder abuse in Chinese communities. Moreover, due to the vast diversities within the Chinese population, we need national and international studies to provide in-depth data on the abuse of older persons. From the policy perspectives, communities, cities, and states should take a critical lead in reducing social isolation, and increasing social networks and companionship for this group of older adults. Incorporating the cultural, social, and community contexts that affect their health and well-being will contribute to the salience of practice and policy impact of prevention, intervention, detection, and reporting of elder abuse for the global Chinese aging population.

II.2

SEVEN POLICY PRIORITIES FOR AN ENHANCED PUBLIC HEALTH RESPONSE TO ELDER ABUSE

Marie-Therese Connolly, J.D., and Ariel Trilling
Woodrow Wilson International Center for Scholars

In 2007, an Institute of Medicine (IOM) workshop took a novel approach to global violence prevention, examining violence horizontally—from war and suicide, to child, gender, sexual, domestic, and elder abuse. At that workshop little was said (and there was not much to say) about research focused on the prevention of elder abuse. Thus, it represents real progress that the IOM, in April 2013, convened a workshop focused on elder abuse and its prevention.

Recent research indicates that elder abuse is a significant and growing problem, victimizing about 1 in 10 Americans age 60 and older living at home, who have and are able to use a phone. For those with limited function, disability, or means to communicate, the numbers appear to be much higher (Acierno et al., 2010; Lifespan of Greater Rochester et al., 2011).[1] Rates of elder abuse rise sharply among people with dementia (Wiglesworth, 2010).[2] In hospitals, nursing homes, and other care settings, research is needed to illuminate current prevalence rates of abuse and neglect; older data and recent cases[3] indicate reason for concern.

As the population ages, caregiver shortages grow, and more people live to an age where they experience physical and cognitive incapacity, the number of people vulnerable to elder abuse will grow. But the problem remains largely hidden. For every case of elder abuse that comes to light, 23 others do not (Lifespan of Greater Rochester et al., 2011). This paper, based on a discussion at the April 2013 IOM workshop, gives an overview of seven policy priorities to enhance the public health response to elder abuse.[4]

Develop Policy to Recognize Elder Abuse as a Public Health Issue

One reason the response to elder abuse lags so far behind comparable issues is that it has not been recognized or treated as a public health issue requiring a public health response. Like other forms of violence, abuse, and neglect, elder abuse is associated with law enforcement, prosecution, social services, and financial issues. Yet it is also a problem that causes premature death and untold suffering, and has major health consequences and costs for individuals, families, and society.

The Centers for Disease Control and Prevention (CDC) and the National Institutes of Health, as well as other public and private entities, have spent billions of dollars to develop a public health response to child abuse and domestic violence. The knowledge and infrastructure relating to elder abuse lag decades behind. To address this gap and the absence of a public health paradigm to address elder abuse, one should begin by collecting

---

[1] The New York state prevalence study found rates of about 7.6 percent, whereas the Acierno study found rates between 11 and 14 percent. Thus, this report uses "about one in ten."

[2] This study, based on 159 dyads of people with dementia and their caregivers, concluded that 47 percent of people with dementia were abused or neglected. Researchers in this study did not screen for financial exploitation.

[3] See, e.g., United States v. Hauser (NDGA, 2012); United States ex rel. Absher v. Momence Meadows Nursing Ctr., Inc., No. 2:04-cv-02289 (C.D. Ill. Feb. 8, 2013); United States v. United States of America ex rel., Kimball and Juelfs v. Cathedral Rock Corporation, Cathedral Rock Management I, Inc. (EDMO, 2010).

[4] These seven points were originally presented in a brief talk that was given at the IOM workshop on elder abuse and its prevention.

data, doing surveillance, and determining (in a methodologically sound way) what types of prevention and intervention programs are effective. Until this is done, elder abuse will remain in the shadows.

Another aspect of this public health problem is the serious shortage of a workforce trained to identify, address, prevent, and study elder abuse. There are roughly 10 times as many pediatricians (most of them trained about child abuse) as geriatricians (few of whom are trained about elder abuse), and the number of geriatricians is falling even as the patient cohort skyrockets (Eldercare Workforce Alliance, 2013). Few geriatricians have training about elder abuse, and even fewer do research to illuminate the problem (this coincides with a general dearth of academic geriatricians). A subspecialty of experts in child abuse, cross-trained in both pediatrics and forensic pathology, has made a difference in shaping how we respond to the problem. There is no comparable subspecialty of *forensic geriatricians*.

These shortages extend to most fields of health and social service workers focused on aging—including nurses, nurse practitioners, physician assistants, geropsychiatrists, and social workers. To improve the response to elder abuse, it is critical that an adequate workforce is developed—trained in how to identify, address, and prevent the problem, and interested in advancing knowledge about it. For these reasons and more, it is critical to recognize elder abuse as a serious public health issue and allocate resources to it accordingly.

Research Priorities Critical to Inform Policy and Practice Relating to Elder Abuse

Responsibly formulating policy is difficult without good data to inform it. More than a decade ago, the National Academy of Sciences (NAS) noted:

> In [prior reports] the National Research Council was able to map out a comprehensive blueprint for research in the adjacent domains of child mistreatment and intimate partner violence. However, so little is now known about elder mistreatment that it would be premature to draw up a detailed research agenda for this nascent field. . . . Abuse and neglect of older individuals in society breaches a widely embraced moral commitment to protect vulnerable people from harm and to ensure their well-being and security. To carry out this commitment, one cannot rely on good intentions alone. A substantial investment in scientific research . . . is imperative. (NRC, 2003, pp. xiii-xiv)

Scientific research has not yet been funded to fulfill this commitment. Five areas to begin, where egregious gaps in knowledge undermine effective policy development, include intervention, defining success, prevention, data collection, and cost.

Intervention

Given the dearth of intervention research, it is unknown whether the programs in place to address elder abuse actually work, or which approaches are more effective than others. APS, mandatory reporting laws, and multidisciplinary teams are three examples of interventions that are broadly relied on, but whose efficacy remains untested. Data are needed so the field can coalesce around strategies and programs that work best.

Defining Success

In assessing the efficacy of an intervention, we must begin by defining *success*. Elder justice advocates have begun to measure the impact of some programs by assessing whether they increase the numbers of reports to law enforcement, prosecutors, or state agencies. Although such information is useful, it does not tell us whether the client, patient, or victim—the person the program is designed to help—considers the intervention a success. Thus, a critical precursor to developing intervention research is determining how to pinpoint success from the perspective of the target population. For those unable to define success for themselves, alternative ways to measure whether the intervention improved well-being need to be used.

Prevention

The field suffers from a critical lack of data on how to prevent elder abuse. Awareness campaigns can be critical means of prevention, but they must be done right. Before undertaking such a campaign (which requires significant resources), it is critical to determine: What do we want to accomplish? Who is the target audience for the message (e.g., older people, families, caregivers, policy makers, or geriatric or public health communities)? What language and message will resonate with that audience? What is the impact of delivering that message to that audience? (Does delivering that message to that audience actually reduce elder abuse? How? What is the most cost-effective dissemination strategy?) Without careful focus and planning, awareness campaigns easily can fall on deaf ears and waste precious resources.

Data Collection

Collecting data about elder abuse is critical to all aspects of policy development. The child abuse field began collecting data in the 1970s in part because a group of experts convened and worked with key state officials to develop a consensus about which standard data points to collect.

The Assistant Secretary for Planning and Evaluation at the Department of Health and Human Services (HHS) issued a report in March 2010 concluding that it is feasible to collect elder abuse data (Office of the Assistant Secretary for Planning and Evaluation, 2010). Although federal law mandates collection of elder abuse data, the data have not yet been collected, nor does a system in place to do so exist. There is no need to reinvent the wheel. State officials and experts in the relevant areas should be convened to lay a foundation and develop a pilot for this critical and long overdue effort.

Cost

Given the massive cost of health care in this nation, research is needed to calculate the unnecessary economic burden elder abuse adds to it. The current knowledge indicates that elder abuse is a hugely expensive problem costing tens of billions of dollars annually: Victims are four times more likely than non-victims to be admitted to nursing homes (Lachs et al., 2007) and three times more likely to be admitted to hospitals (Dong and Simon, 2013). Taxpayers (primarily through Medicare and Medicaid) foot the lion's share of the bill for those increased care needs. Financial exploitation also has serious economic consequences, leading to higher rates of dual eligibility and increased reliance on other public programs (Gunther, 2011); for example, victims whose assets are depleted are more likely to need public housing. In addition, elder abuse leads to economic losses for employers, businesses, families, and individuals.

Elder abuse tips over otherwise autonomous older people's lives, causing increased dependence. Victims who do not go to facilities are likely to become more dependent on informal caregivers. Voluminous data have shown that caregiving takes a huge health and financial toll on caregivers (MetLife Mature Market Institute, 2011). This is another massive, uncalculated downstream cost of elder abuse. As policy makers grapple with how to reduce the price of health care, they need data about the many ways in which elder abuse drains an overburdened system with avoidable costs.

Policy Opportunity: Translate What We Do Know into Practice

Amidst the dire gaps in knowledge, there are some data about elder abuse. Yet these data are too rarely applied (Acierno et al., 2010).[5] For example, older people with good social supports and services are known to be less likely to become victims of elder abuse, neglect, and financial exploitation than those who lack those resources (Acierno et al., 2010). Yet effective

---

[5] This is not only a problem in the elder abuse field. Atul Gawande has noted that, in medicine, "good ideas take an appallingly long time to trickle down."

coordination is not assured or adequately promoted between (1) those in the elder abuse field and (2) the entities that provide or coordinate social support, including those in the aging network, caregiving field, care managers and planners, Alzheimer's and dementia policy makers and programs, faith-based organizations, and home- and community-based services.

Second, APS workers and others charged with making decisions about when and how to intervene in the face of alleged elder abuse often have insufficient training or outdated tools to decide whether and when to seek expert capacity assessment of the person they are trying to help. Though capacity will remain a challenging issue, the data that do exist could be used more effectively, and APS could ensure correct use of the right instruments to inform and enhance the decisions of APS workers and others (Karlawish, 2013).

Third, health, social service, and law enforcement responders often encounter older people with bruises and must decide whether those bruises are reason for concern. Research is now available about such *forensic markers* to help responders distinguish between inflicted and accidental bruises and determine whether a case should be referred for further investigation (Mosqueda et al., 2005). But the bruising data are not well disseminated, so many people who could use the data do not.

Resources and Policy: Chicken and Egg

The biggest reason there is so little research to guide elder justice policy, and so few researchers do elder abuse research, is the dearth of funds to support such research. The General Accountability Office (GAO) highlighted the issue in March 2011. The GAO found the following funding amount to elder abuse research (in 2009):

- National Institute on Aging (NIA): $1.1 million, which is about 1/1000th of its budget;
- CDC: $50,000, which is 0.0008 percent of its budget (CDC has spent millions and been a leader on child abuse and domestic violence issues); and
- National Institute of Justice (NIJ), the Department of Justice (DOJ) research arm: $450,000 of its funds, plus other DOJ dollars, totaling $1.2 million.

The total—$2.35 million for elder abuse research (as last calculated by GAO in 2009)—is a tiny fraction of federal funds spent annually for research on analogous issues (GAO, 2011).

The same disparity appears in the distribution of victim assistance funds, relatively few of which are allocated to older victims or to better understand how to address older victims' needs (often different from those of younger crime victims). The same GAO study found that the Office for Victims of Crime expended only 0.5 percent of its budget on older victims (GAO, 2011). One possible reason for this disparity is that unlike victims of child abuse and sexual and domestic violence, some of whom can and do speak out very effectively, few elder abuse victims are able to do so.

The dearth of resources available to address elder abuse diminishes the quality of the response to the problem, undermines policy development, and impedes efforts to recruit people to the field. Allocation of resources is one way societies, agencies, foundations, and other funders show what issues they believe to be important. Young researchers and practitioners carefully observe such funding trends and are understandably hesitant to choose a field that lacks priority or resources. The relationship between resources and policy is circular. Policy helps determine where to send resources. Resources fund research and programs that inform policy.

Implement Law and Develop Policy Infrastructure

The Child Abuse Prevention and Treatment Act and the Violence Against Women Act (VAWA), with other laws, created offices at HHS and DOJ that for decades have assured leadership, research, funding, programmatic efforts, and policy development to redress child abuse and domestic violence. Such offices are a low-cost, high-impact way to bring sustained attention, coordination, momentum, and more effective use of existing resources relating to elder abuse.

Creation of offices and other infrastructure promoting ongoing, thoughtful policy attention to elder abuse was a central catalyst for the Elder Justice Act (EJA), the first comprehensive federal law to address elder abuse. First introduced in 2002, the law took 8 years to pass. Its 2010 enactment was met with great anticipation. As of 2013, however, the law has not been funded and, in most part, not implemented. The section that would have created an office was not part of the law that was enacted.

Develop a Political Constituency

Why has a law that once had broad bipartisan support not been funded or implemented? Why have elder abuse concerns not been better integrated into existing programs relating to aging, disability, health, law, caregiving, and consumer protection? Why are public leaders and the public not more engaged in an issue with a profound impact on the lives of millions of people? Why do good ideas, good programs, important research, and promising innovations remain isolated in pockets, rarely translating into policy or systems change? The answer in large part is that the elder justice movement lacks nearly every aspect of a political constituency—grassroots and grasstops networks, strategic policy development, strategic legal action and communication plans, diverse constituencies joining to address the problem, and high-profile champions.

The initial enactment and recent reauthorization of VAWA illustrate the importance of a strong political constituency (including the critical role of a high-level champion like Vice President Joe Biden, first in the Senate, then in the White House). The National Alzheimer's Project Act (NAPA) provides another example in a related field. NAPA was enacted in 2011 after the EJA, but its Federal Advisory Committee was promptly convened (in 2011). Compare this with the EJA's Advisory Board that has yet to be convened, though its report was due to Congress in March 2011. The EJA-created Elder Justice Coordinating Council finally met for the first time in 2012 with participation of HHS Secretary Kathleen Sebelius and Attorney General Eric Holder. The field is awaiting the results of that federal coordination.

Promote Innovation

While we were working on the EJA Judy Salerno, then Deputy Director of NIA, provided a critical piece of advice. *Support innovation.* Not all people who have great potentially life-changing ideas can get them funded by entities like NIA, NIJ, or elite foundations. We thus included a section in the EJA that would have created an innovation fund. Coast to coast, people create new programs, try new approaches, and think up new ideas based on their experience and expertise. We need to find better ways to harness that innovation, to figure out which innovations work and replicate them. Unfortunately, the innovation section did not find its way into the final EJA, but there are other paths to this goal. By funding the recent prevention grants, HHS has offered such an opportunity using another vehicle.

A critical innovation is the proliferation of different types of multidisciplinary teams, such as elder abuse (forensic) centers (by whatever name) and financial abuse specialist teams at the federal, state, and local levels all over the country. The EJA-created federal Elder Justice Coordinating Council is also such a team. These teams promote development of new ways to respond to elder abuse within disciplines, and allow groups of people and disciplines to innovate new ways of doing things *together*. Although it is an article of faith that multidisciplinary teams (MDTs) are effective, there are many models and many challenges, and little data to tell us what works best. Taking a more analytic approach to evaluating them could elicit valuable information to those guiding and forming such teams and to policy makers shaping policy related to them.

Countless billions of dollars have been spent to lengthen life. The time has come to honor that *widely embraced moral commitment* cited by the

NRC in 2003 and make a meaningful research and policy investment to enhance well-being in the years we have gained.

II.3

ELDER NEGLECT: THE STATE OF THE SCIENCE

Terry T. Fulmer, Ph.D., R.N.
Bouve College of Health Sciences, Northeastern University

XinQi Dong, M.D., M.P.H.
Chinese Health, Aging, and Policy Program,
Rush Institute for Healthy Aging
Rush University Medical Center

Elder Neglect Review: The Research Overview

Inadequate progress has been made in our understanding of elder mistreatment and particularly the subtype of elder neglect. Three areas of investigation in elder mistreatment research have made advances in knowledge, improving our understanding in areas including the incidence and prevalence of elder mistreatment (Cisler et al., 2010), self-neglect (Dyer et al., 2007; Dong et al., 2009, 2010a,b), and resident-to-resident mistreatment (Lachs et al., 2007). However, there continues to be negligible advancement in our understanding of neglect of older people by other individuals. The purpose of this paper is to review studies that have data specific to neglect by others, document trends in the data, underscore the concern related to the limited number of scientists engaged in this important area, and begin to determine how intervention studies can be developed to reduce and eliminate neglect to older individuals. Several investigators have documented that elder neglect is a potentially fatal syndrome and that of all individuals in the elder mistreatment category, those in the neglect category have significant risk for morbidity and mortality. A systematic review of all research databases was conducted to ascertain the state of the science related to elder neglect, and those papers with original data are reported here. The study of neglect appears to have three main approaches: examination of cases using prospective longitudinal cohort studies against other databases, screening for cases in practice settings, and postmortem analysis.

Elder neglect has been defined by the National Research Council as "an omission by responsible caregivers that constitutes neglect under applicable federal or state law" (NRC, 2003, p. 39). Others have defined it as "the refusal or failure by those responsible to provide food, shelter, health care, or protection for a vulnerable elder" (National Center on Elder Abuse, 2013).

Elder Neglect Literature Review

Early studies with data on neglect include the elder abuse and neglect findings from *Three Model Projects* (Godkin et al., 1989), in which a case comparison study was completed that examined 62 individuals from Worcester, Massachusetts, and 65 from Boston, Massachusetts. Active neglect was found in 20 percent of the cases. Neglect had the strongest relationship to dependency needs of the victims and neglect cases had significant problems for cognitive and physical functioning. Individuals who were neglected were less likely to be burdensome and stressful, but caregivers had significant stressors in their own lives.

In a 1984 study, Fulmer and Cahill conducted elder mistreatment assessments on all patients arriving at a busy emergency room using screening by the nurses on that floor who had been trained to use the particular elder assessment instrument (Fulmer and Cahill, 1984). In this work, investigators chose a "good, fair, poor" scale to elicit nursing concerns related to suspected elder mistreatment. This strategy failed in that in the majority of cases, nurses selected the midline (fair) and were reticent to make judgments about suspected mistreatment. Subsequently, a body of work used a 4-point scale of "very good, good, poor, very poor" and was found to be much preferred in that nurses would lean to the positive or negative in order to better understand suspected cases of elder abuse and neglect. In each of these screens, neglect was by far the most predominant selected category (over abuse, neglect, exploitation, or abandonment).

Pillemer and Finkelhor (1988) conducted the first large-scale random sample survey of elder mistreatment involving 2,020 elderly persons from Boston. Of those individuals, 63 persons were maltreated and 7 out of 63 came out of the category of neglect. Thirty-two per 1,000 older individuals in this study were labeled as mistreated, with 4 in 1,000 labeled as neglected. The perpetrators in the neglect cases were husband–wife (29 percent), daughter–mother (29 percent), and other (42 percent), which is a strong indicator that the phenomena was not well explained in this study. The most common characteristics of neglect in this study included victims who were female, were divorced, had a spouse and children, were in poor health, and were without a helper. Neglect victims were commonly in poor health and reported that they did not have close contacts on whom they could rely. This work has proven extremely valuable in anchoring subsequent research.

Fulmer and Ashley examined 107 cases of suspected neglect and referred to an elder mistreatment team compared with 146 non-referred cases (Fulmer and Ashley, 1989). An expert panel was asked to select indicators of neglect from the Elder Assessment Instrument (EAI). Nine neglect indicators were selected. A factor analysis of those items indicated that nutritional deficits, alterations in skin integrity, and alterations in elimination patterns were the three major clusters constituting neglect symptoms.

In a study of patients presenting to the emergency department over a 6-month period (Fulmer and Degutis, 1992; Fulmer et al., 1992), 3,153 recorded visits for older adults represented 1,975 older individuals (a significant recidivism to the emergency room). Of those, 56 percent were female with a mean age of 76.5 years. The group was predominantly white. Of those included in the group, 126 individuals (4 percent) were recorded as having some sort of elder mistreatment. Of those, 55 percent were recorded as neglect, further evidence that neglect is the most prevalent category of mistreatment. In that study, associations with the outcome of mistreatment include non-white, not married, and without insurance, as well as with some form of delirium or dementia. These associations with mistreatment represent vulnerable older adults. Associations with abuse and neglect included those who were non-white and non-married. However, it is interesting that neglect was associated with delirium and dementia, while abuse was not. Again, this speaks to the vulnerable older adult.

Using a prospective longitudinal cohort database (Lachs et al., 1996; Harrell et al., 2002), Lachs and others compared APS records and determined that in a group of 2,812 individuals, 184 cases were suspected of some form of mistreatment, with 81 cases substantiated. Of those, 30 individuals (64 percent) experienced neglect by another party. In a follow-up study on mortality of elder mistreatment, Lachs and colleagues (1997) documented that of 176 older adults seen by APS over 9 years, 30 (17 percent) were for cases of neglect.

In an emergency room pilot feasibility study conducted over a 3-week period, 180 patients ages 70 and older were screened using the EAI to determine how well it worked in busy practice environments. Of the 180 patients who met the age criteria, 36 agreed to be screened and 7 screened positive for neglect. The purpose of this pilot was to determine if nurses were able to screen with accuracy versus an elder mistreatment team. There was 70 percent accuracy for detecting neglect between the nurses and the expert team (Fulmer et al., 2000).

Pavlik and colleagues (2001) used a statewide database to describe the case reports received in 1997 by the Texas Department of Protective and Regulatory Services-Adult Protective Services Division (TDPRS-APS). They documented more than 62,000 allegations of adult mistreatment and neglect. Neglect accounted for 80 percent of the allegations. The incidence of cases in the TDPRS-APS increased sharply after age 65. The prevalence was 1,310 individuals/100,000 for all abuse types. Dyer et al. (2007) asked APS workers to describe elder neglect in an effort to define a working case definition. Using a structured interview, the authors asked APS workers in Texas to identify indicators of elder neglect that they see in practice. The most common indicator (36 percent) was cited to be derangement in the client's environment. This involved the condition of the home, including debris and food left on the floors, as well as the outside environment of the home. The second most identified factor (18.4 percent) was personal hygiene. The workers were also asked to define both self-neglect and caregiver neglect. The majority distinguished caregiver neglect as simply having a caregiver present. The study concluded that elder neglect could be described by deficiencies in environmental cleanliness, cognition, and personal hygiene. Physicians and other home care workers should consider the home environment as well as personal hygiene when screening for elder neglect (Harrell et al., 2002; Bitondo Dyer et al., 2005).

International Studies

Chokkanathan and Lee conducted a probability study in urban India to determine cases of mistreatment. Of 400 older adults surveyed, 56 (14 percent) reported mistreatment, and of the 14 percent, 4.3 percent reported neglect versus 5 percent physical abuse. This again underscores the presence of neglect across cultures (Chokkanathan and Lee, 2005). Oh et al. (2006) studied the prevalence of elder abuse and neglect in South Korea, and they interviewed 15,230 adults ages 65 and older. The percentage of older adults who experienced any type of elder abuse was 6.3 percent. An abusive act was defined as occurring more than once and occurring more than two or three times per month. Of participants, 2.4 percent reported neglect. Furthermore, they identified the main abuser for each type of abuse. For neglect, the main abuser was identified as the daughter-in-law at 38 percent.

Dong et al. (2007) investigated the prevalence of elder abuse and neglect in an urban Chinese population. A cross-sectional study was performed in a major urban medical center in Nanjing, China. A total of 412 participants completed the survey and 145 participants (35 percent) screened positive for elder abuse and neglect. The mean age of the victims was 69 years, and 59 percent were male. Caregiver neglect was the most common form of abuse, followed by financial exploitation, psychological abuse, physical abuse, sexual abuse, and abandonment. Thirty-six percent of the victims suffered multiple forms of abuse and neglect. In the logistic regression analyses of the data, female gender, lower education, and lower income were demographic risk factors associated with elder abuse and neglect. Dong and colleagues reported that a better understanding of these and additional risk factors associated with elder abuse and neglect in older Chinese people is needed. They further examined depression as a risk factor for elder abuse and neglect in this population. Depression was assessed using the Geriatric Depression Scale and direct questions were asked regarding abuse and neglect experienced by the elderly since the age of 60; 412 patients completed the survey. The mean age of the participants was 70; 34 percent were female. Depression was found in 12 percent of the participants, and elder abuse and neglect were found in 35 percent. After multiple logistic regression, feeling of dissatisfaction with life (OR, 2.92; 95 percent CI, 1.51-5.68, $p < 0.001$), often being bored (OR, 2.91; CI, 1.53-5.55, $p < 0.001$), often feeling helpless (OR, 2.79; CI, 1.35-5.76, $p < 0.001$), and feeling worthless (OR, 2.16; CI, 1.10-4.22, $p < 0.001$) were associated with increased risk of elder abuse and neglect. Multiple logistic regression modeling showed that depression is independently associated with elder abuse and neglect (OR, 3.26; CI, 1.49-7.10, $p < 0.003$). One limitation of this study is that there was not sufficient power to clearly separate out abuse from neglect and the two forms of mistreatment were reported together. However, these findings suggest that depression is a significant risk factor associated with elder abuse and neglect among Chinese elderly. Subsequent studies should address the two forms independently (Dong, 2008).

The prevalence of physical and financial abuse among Turkish elderly in two different socioeconomic strata was reported. Keskinoglu et al. (2007) selected a district of low socioeconomic status, and documented physical and financial abuse prevalence was 1.5 and 2.5 percent, respectively, while among the elderly in the district of high socioeconomic status, it was 2 and 0.3 percent, respectively. However, the prevalence of elder neglect in the two districts was 27.4 and 11.2 percent, respectively. Prevalence of neglect was associated with infrequent contact with relatives, little or no income, and fewer years of education among the elderly in the low socioeconomic district. In the high socioeconomic district, neglect was associated with fewer years of education, poor health status, and having chronic status. They concluded that the prevalence of abuse among the elderly living in the two different districts was low, but nearly one-fifth of elderly people were exposed to neglect. Here, again the phenomenon of neglect holds up as construct internationally. This is important because it has been postulated that neglect may be identified in some cultures and not in others. However, there is a growing body of evidence that the construct of neglect holds across cultures.

Clinical Assessment Approaches: Use of Autopsies

Obviously, neglect takes place in the context of the older adult and some other person. Using a dyadic approach would allow the investigators to interview both the elder and the caregiver (Fulmer et al., 2005a). Fulmer and colleagues (2005a) examined vulnerability and risk profiling for elder neglect. In that study, 5,159 older adults were approached for inclusion and 3,669 were screened and recruited through five emergency departments in New York City and Tampa, Florida. Of those screened, 405 met the inclusion criteria (11 percent) and agreed to participate. Of the 405 older adults and caregivers who were eligible to participate, 165 (41 percent) completed the face-to-face, in-home interview.

In all, the demographics of the neglect versus the non-neglect groups were the same, except that the neglect group had fewer people living in the home ($p < .04$), were more likely to be Hispanic or Latino by self-report ($p < .02$), had a health problem that limited activities ($p < .05$), and were more likely to be Medicare recipients ($p < .03$). Caregivers of the neglect group were more likely to be Hispanic or Latino by self-report ($p < .04$), were less likely to have health problems that required a doctor's attention ($p < .02$), and were less likely to be on Medicare ($p < .01$). The mean ages of the two caregiver groups were not significantly different. The data supported the idea that vulnerable older adults who have cognitive impairment have increased functional needs and were more likely to suffer from neglect. Furthermore, the absence of social support, childhood trauma, as well as the personality trait "openness" on the NEO personality inventory scale (McCrae and Costa, 1987) created the association with the neglect outcome (Fulmer et al., 2005b). In another study that enrolled patients from busy primary care clinics, including a dental clinic, older adults were screened with the EAI, and the prevalence of mistreatment was 4 percent, with neglect as the most prevalent subcategory. In that study, associations were documented between cognitive function and caregiver neglect. Furthermore, this study demonstrated that elder neglect can be screened for and examined in busy primary care clinics (Russell et al., 2012).

Akaza et al. (2003) documented neglect and abuse by examining 15 autopsy cases in Gifu Prefecture, Japan, between 1990 and 2000. Using a retrospective approach of all the cases in which the victim was 65 years or older and autopsied, 15 victims were classified as elder abuse victims: 5 men and 10 women. The victims ranged in age from 66 to 87 years (mean age, 74.5 years). The types of abuse were as follows: physical abuse, 13 cases; emotional abuse, 5 cases; neglect, 4 cases; and financial abuse, 3 cases. In eight cases, the victims were subjected to two or more types of abuse. The cause of death of the victims varied with the type of abuse. In the physical abuse cases, subdural hemorrhage was the most common cause, followed by other violence-related deaths and hypothermia. In the neglect cases, the victims died of either starvation or suffocation after the aspiration of food into the airway. In the domestic abuse cases, one of the victim's sons was the most common perpetrator, and little or no income was considered to be a risk factor for perpetrators. In the neglect cases, dementia and difficulty in performing activities of daily living were considered to be risk factors for victims, in addition to living in social isolation.

Collins and Presnell (2007) also used autopsy cases in a retrospective review of individuals 65 years and older over a 20-year period, and determined that eight cases of suspected neglect resulted in death. The causes of death included sepsis due to extreme dehydration and severe decubitus ulcers. Unfortunately there were no follow-up studies to this analysis, but the work and the approach represent another important way to research neglect and its potential outcomes. Interestingly, the dehydration and decubitus ulcers often occur due to the conditions of nutritional status and skin integrity (Fulmer and Ashley, 1989).

In another example of postmortem analysis, Shields and colleagues (2004) conducted a retrospective 10-year study of elder abuse and neglect cases in Kentucky and Indiana. They reviewed postmortem records and also reviewed examinations under the Clinical Forensic Medicine Program. The authors described 74 postmortem cases, of which 22 deaths were suspicious for neglect. Of those, the most common cause of death was bronchopneumonia. They identified 22 living victims, and of those 3 were identified as suffering from neglect. The authors concluded that a multidisciplinary team approach is crucial to identifying cases of elder neglect, and the importance of the forensic team and Medical Examiner's office should not be ignored (Shields et al., 2004).

National Elder Mistreatment Study: United States

In 2010, a study was published that has set the stage for future research, and has created a new baseline for research in the field. Acierno et al. (2010), in the National Elder Mistreatment Study from 2010, used a definition of neglect as "failing to meet the following needs: transportation, household needs (i.e., cooking and cleaning), taking care of financial matters, and obtaining medication." They reported on a representative sample using random digit dialing across geographic strata, analyzing 5,777 respondents. They reported a prevalence of 4.6 percent for emotional abuse, 1.6 percent for physical abuse, 0.6 percent for sexual abuse, 5.1 percent for potential neglect, and 5.2 percent for financial abuse (Acierno et al., 2010). Approximately 1 in 10 respondents reported some mistreatment in the past year. They found that the risk for potential neglect was predicted by low income, lack of social support, racial minority status, and poor health. In general, the study found that the most significant predictors of abuse and neglect were low social support and exposure to a traumatic event. This aligns with data from a Fulmer study in 2005 (Fulmer et al., 2005a). The associations between cognitive function and elder abuse and neglect were documented previously by others using the Chicago Health and Aging Project database (Dong et al., 2012c). Neglect is second only to financial abuse in this report and clearly these data should trigger investigators to respond to the important unanswered questions on the subject of neglect by others.

Summary of the Evidence

In summary, evidence since the 1980s would indicate that the overall prevalence of mistreatment is approximately 4 to 10 percent, and neglect is the most prevalent subcategory. Neglect can have dire clinical consequences and increase the mortality in older adults. Few investigators have taken on the topic of neglect by others in a caregiving relationship, and the need for additional research on this topic is clear. Assessing for elder neglect in the clinical setting should be a standard of care. Of concern, Cooper et al. (2008) conducted a systematic review of the prevalence of elder abuse and neglect using multiple databases and independent raters and identified 49 studies meeting the inclusion criteria, of which only 7 used measures for which reliability and validity had been assessed and established. Clinicians need guidance in addressing this phenomenon and clinical assessment instrumentation must improve. Several of the current instruments are either flawed psychometrically or require disrobing of the patient for full assessment, which is impractical in many settings.

Likely, most cases of neglect go undetected, and currently we have no intervention studies, except for Wiglesworth et al.'s (2006) work related to bruising and Dyer et al.'s (1999) team approach to cases of abuse and neglect. To this point, research on elder neglect has predominantly taken the form of documenting the presence in longitudinal cohort studies, and screening for incidence and prevalence of neglect and reviewing autopsy cases. We argue that it is essential for investigators to take on the extremely challenging topic of elder neglect by trusted others, whether they are formal or informal caregivers, and begin to understand how we can create intervention strategies to prevent neglect. By doing so, it is highly likely that we can decrease the morbidity and mortality associated with this phenomenon.

II.4

NATIVE ELDER MISTREATMENT

Lori L. Jervis, Ph.D.
Department of Anthropology and Center for Applied Research,
University of Oklahoma

Introduction

This paper examines elder mistreatment among American Indians/ Alaskan Natives (AIs/ANs). To date, only limited empirical research has been conducted on this phenomenon due to the sensitivity of the topic, cultural nuances around what constitutes mistreatment, practical challenges involved in carrying out research among the numerous sovereign tribes across the United States, and lack of targeted funding devoted to this issue. Although the knowledge base on Native elder mistreatment is sparse, the small studies that have been conducted are sufficient to suggest directions for future investigation.

Prevalence and Risk Factors

The prevalence of elder mistreatment in the AI/AN population is unknown. To date, a large-scale, population-based prevalence study of Native elder abuse or neglect has not been carried out. Several factors complicate the possibility of prevalence studies among AIs/ANs. Perhaps the most notable of these is the great number and diversity of Native groups, which include 566 federally recognized AI tribes and AN villages, more than 64 state-recognized tribes, and 14 tribes with active petitions with the Bureau of Indian Affairs for recognition (Bureau of Indian Affairs, 2013). Federally recognized AI tribes and AN corporations are sovereign nations, each of which has its own approaches to dealing with researchers who wish to work with them. Moreover, the great diversity found among the Native population makes it difficult to adapt items or generalize across so many cultural groups/nations.

While a large-scale prevalence study has not yet been conducted, several smaller studies give a preliminary indication of prevalence in select settings. Medical record reviews of 550 AI/AN urban primary care clinic patients ages 50 and older found that 10 percent were definitely or probably physically abused. In 88.8 percent of cases where the gender of the abuser(s) was known, the victim was female and the perpetrator male (Buchwald et al., 2000). Those who were abused were significantly more likely to be female ($p < 0.001$), younger ($p < 0.001$), depressed ($p < 0.001$), and dependent on others for food ($p < 0.05$). Authorities were notified in only 31 percent of cases of definite abuse. In a study of 100 AIs ages 60 and older (both reservation and metropolitan), more than half (53 percent) were found to be at risk of mistreatment based on either the Hwalek-Sengstock Elder Abuse Screening Test (HS-EAST) (Neale et al., 1990, 1991) or the Native Elder Life Scale-Financial Exploitation or Neglect measures (Jervis et al., 2013).

A study of 152 health and human service providers to Navajo elders found that neglect and financial exploitation were considered the most common types of abuse (Brown et al., 1990). Physically abusive caregivers tended to be younger, be unemployed, have more personal problems, live with victims, have other responsibilities, and be less likely to receive help from others. Having any kind of income was a risk factor for physical and psychological abuse, as were shared caregiving arrangements and mental confusion (Brown, 1989). A study of risk factors among two different groups of Plains Indians found that higher levels of abuse were found on the more isolated and impoverished reservation (Maxwell and Maxwell, 1992). Although it is not yet clear how economic conditions and elder mistreatment intersect, the poverty within many Native communities may increase risk by fostering economic dependency of the young on the relatively stable elderly (Brown, 1989).

Cultural Conceptions of Abuse

Physical abuse seems relatively "straightforward" compared to many other forms of mistreatment (e.g., psychological abuse, financial exploitation, neglect). After all, what cultural group would condone physically harming an elder? As the ethnographic record demonstrates, however, elders are treated in a variety of ways across the globe—which includes great esteem and extensive support at one extreme to profound ridicule and even homicide on the other (Barker, 2009; Glascock, 2009). Mistreatment is, in fact, a culturally relative issue in the sense that cultural groups have their own notions of "right" and "wrong" treatment of elders. In the United States, what appears to be abusive to the majority population may not be interpreted that way by ethnic minority elders themselves (Rittman et al., 1999). Likewise, what appears to be abusive to Native elders may not be seen as abusive by the general population. Particular cultural groups may also have unique ways of describing or categorizing abuse. For instance, the term "spiritual abuse" has been used among some AIs to apply to situations such as elders being denied access to ceremonies or to traditional healing (NIEJI, 2013). Notions of severity may also differ among ethnic/cultural groups. In a comparison of perceptions of elder abuse among 944 AIs, European Americans, and African Americans using case vignettes, similar notions of abuse across groups were found (Hudson and Carlson, 1999). However, AIs classified the greatest number of vignettes as abusive and severe. It is crucial to understand how individuals and communities experiencing mistreatment conceptualize it because this ultimately affects many aspects of how these behaviors will be responded to and managed within communities.

The Shielding American Indian Elders (SAIE) project[6] examined cultural understandings of elder mistreatment among 100 AIs ages 60 and older from a Northern Plains reservation and a South–Central metropolitan area using a Community Based Participatory Research approach (Jervis et al., 2013). The project's qualitative component examined participants' ideas about what it meant to be treated well and poorly by family (self-defined because "family" in Native communities frequently encompasses individuals who are not biological relatives). Good treatment emerged as a complex mixture of being taken care of, having one's needs met, and being respected. Poor treatment, on the other hand, was defined as financial exploitation, neglect, and lack of respect (Jervis et al., in preparation). Respect was a crucial component of what it meant to be treated well, while disrespect was largely equated with abuse.

Cultural subtleties about mistreatment are especially pronounced when considering financial exploitation. In the SAIE project (as well as in other formal and informal conversations with Native communities), financial exploitation has proven to be a highly salient issue, evoking much concern about its presumed escalation. Yet, the question of what exactly constitutes financial exploitation and what factors propel it is far from resolved. While theft constituted the bulk of financial exploitation in SAIE, other variants that are woven into the fabric of Native life were noted. For instance, exploitive child care is often offered as a prime example of elder mistreatment by community members, yet it remains difficult for Native elders themselves to differentiate it from culturally normative and esteemed childcare (Jervis et al., in preparation). That this might constitute a "gray area" is understandable because close grandparent–grandchild relationships that include childcare (and where children may provide eldercare) are quite common among AIs/ANs (Schweitzer, 1999; Jervis et al., 2010), as are cultural values that emphasize familial (and financial) interdependence (Red Horse, 1983). Yet, in situations of pervasive poverty, dislocation, diminished health, and overcrowded tribal housing, traditional values and norms may be altered in such a way that they act to the detriment of elders (and sometimes to the

---

[6] Funding for the Shielding American Indian Elders Project was provided by the National Institute of Aging (1 R21 AG030686-01, Jervis PI). The Shielding American Indian Elders Team includes David Baldridge, Jan Beals, Connie Bremner, Dedra Buchwald, John Compton, Alexandra Fickenscher, William Foote, Julie Holden, Yvonne M. Jackson, Lisa James, Chebon Kernell, Crystal LoudHawk-Hedgepeth, Spero M. Manson, Traci McClellan-Sorell, Lisa Nerenberg, Emily Matt Salois, William Sconzert-Hall, Bessie Smith, Charlene Smith, and Gloria Tallbull.

children in the household as well). Indeed, it may be a mistake to assume that Native elder abuse is an isolated dyadic issue. Because of the centrality of the extended family among AIs/ANs (Red Horse, 1983, 1997), elder mistreatment should be viewed in the context of the larger family system, and the possibility of child abuse/neglect and/or interpersonal violence should be considered as well.

Law Enforcement and APS

The U.S. colonization of AIs/ANs has resulted in disrupted cultural, economic, and kinship systems, which no doubt affects the way in which elders are treated (Jervis et al., 2003; National Indian Council on Aging, 2004; Jervis and AI-SUPERPFP Team, 2009). In the contemporary era, those responsible for dealing with Native elder mistreatment face many challenges due to lack of resources coupled with the unique legal, jurisdictional, and law enforcement issues related to AIs/ANs' sovereign nation status (Biolsi, 2001, 2005). Victims of violence may feel the police or judicial system cannot help them, and therefore may be reluctant to seek help. Tribal police forces are often stretched thin in terms of economic resources and personnel, often with a small number of officers covering large reservations and rural areas (Wakeling et al., 2001). Geographic isolation from police and social services may heighten fear of retaliation. In smaller communities, it is often a reality that the elder will come into contact with the perpetrator/family of perpetrator even after abuse is reported. Underreporting of crime has also been attributed to shame/humiliation and the longstanding distrust of law enforcement authorities among AIs/ANs (Wakeling et al., 2001).

Complicating this picture is the fact that a large number of tribes do not yet have laws focused on elder abuse (NIEJI, 2013). In addition, many tribes have no APS of their own, necessitating that cases be investigated by the state in which they are located, which may not be equipped to handle the cultural subtleties involved. Some tribes that do have APS are staffed by volunteers who may not be able to devote their full attention to the cases they encounter. These factors may contribute to the sense that the risks of reporting mistreatment are not worth the possible benefits. Elders and family members may be additionally motivated by the desire to maintain a sense of privacy around their family's "business" or to keep the kin group together; concern about losing grandchildren; the fear of ending up in a nursing home; and/or a sense of responsibility for the abuser, for whom the elder may be a caregiver. When considered as a whole, it is not surprising that Native elder mistreatment so often goes unreported.

Future Directions

The empirical research thus far indicates a small but growing knowledge base with respect to AI/AN elder mistreatment. Several research directions have been identified that are especially worthy of future examination. In terms of determining prevalence, the ideal would be a population-based prevalence study that could shed light on how widespread elder mistreatment actually is among AIs/ANs. However, conceptualization studies are also necessary to better understand elder and community perceptions. With respect to this latter line of research, of particular importance are the following questions: Where is the breaking point for tolerating mistreatment, both from an individual and a community perspective? Perceived severity is important to understand, especially with respect to the various types of mistreatment. For instance, is financial exploitation worthy of intervention? Are all types of financial exploitation seen as equal? How about other forms of mistreatment? Where does the line get crossed such that various types of actions are believed to be necessary (e.g., telling a friend or relative what is going on, notifying APS, calling the police, etc.)? Another important area of exploration concerns the informal behaviors/actions people engage in when encountering mistreated elders in their communities. This might involve their willingness to involve themselves or attempts to circumvent systems that are seen as inadequate (e.g., dealing with mistreatment within/between families). Research that attempts to understand what actions/systems various actors deem desirable, useful, futile, etc., would be potentially fruitful.

Although it might seem that sexual and physical abuse are the most clear-cut forms of mistreatment, in fact the resources to deal even with these crimes are generally inadequate. It is exceedingly rare to hear of a successfully prosecuted case. Given these issues, alternatives to the existing criminal justice model, such as restorative justice (Holkup et al., 2007), should be explored. Research that can inform prevention, detection, mediation, and interventions for all types of mistreatment among AIs/ANs are called for at this juncture, especially given the challenges that many Native communities face with respect to law enforcement, APS, and the criminal justice system.

II.5

ELDER FINANCIAL ABUSE

Ronald Long, J.D.
Regulatory Affairs, Wells Fargo Advisors, LLC

Introduction

The scourge of elder financial abuse has received considerable attention from many over the past few years.[7] The GAO (2012) cited it as "an epidemic with society-wide repercussions." Almost by definition, the challenge for financial services companies is more direct and urgent as they are often holding "the keys to the kingdom" on which the abusers have set their sights. To respond to this daunting task, individual banks and brokerage firms, and the financial services industry as a whole, have undertaken a number of initiatives to detect, deter, and respond to the elder financial abuse events they are seeing more of every day. This paper outlines the efforts of one firm, Wells Fargo Advisors (WFA),[8] which has created infrastructure, initiatives, and systems designed to detect, deter, and report third-party elder financial abuse.[9]

The Wells Fargo Advisors Inventory

A major part of the WFA effort in addressing elder financial abuse flows from the stark realization that what are generally described as reasons the elderly are targets precisely overlays the WFA client base. Elders are targeted for abuse because, as a group, they tend to possess more money. Older Americans are 47 percent wealthier than younger Americans (Censky, 2011). Persons over age 50 control more than 70 percent of the nation's wealth (National Committee for the Prevention of Elder Abuse, 2008), and 81 percent of households headed by people 65 and older own

---

[7] See http://www.nij.gov/topics/crime/elder-abuse.

[8] WFA is a non-bank affiliate of Wells Fargo & Company ("Wells Fargo"), a diversified financial services company providing banking, insurance, investments, mortgage, and consumer and commercial finance across the United States and internationally. Wells Fargo has $1.3 trillion in assets and more than 265,000 team members across 80-plus businesses. The elder financial abuse work is a corporate-wide initiative, but for ease of discussion, this paper will focus primarily on the effort in WFA. The paper will use the terms "WFA" and "Wells Fargo" interchangeably.

[9] As a part of the highly regulated U.S. securities industry, WFA uses and relies on several layers of protection against any employee who may mistreat an elder client. The firm's compliance systems and its federal, state, and private regulators all have this rarer issue uppermost in their missions. Accordingly, this paper will focus on the instances of preventing third-party elder financial abuse and essentially self-abuse through the client's declining capacity.

their homes (*Washington Post*, 2012). Households headed by people 75 or older have the highest median net wealth of any age group (U.S. Census Bureau, 2012).

The statistics for WFA clients are almost mirror images of these national statistics. The majority of the $1.2 trillion in assets held by WFA are owned by clients who are over 60 years old. Even more, many of our clients are actually retired or soon to be retired, so safeguarding their nest eggs is even more critical because these clients will have no opportunity to find new employment income to make up for losses suffered due to elder abuse. With an estimated 10,000 persons turning 65 every day for the next 20 years, the potential for a WFA client to become a victim of elder financial abuse is increasing dramatically.

Training

An initial decision for a financial services company that desires to handle elder financial abuse is simply to raise internal awareness of this issue. For example, Wells Fargo requires annual training of the majority of its employees. At WFA, computer-based training on "Reporting Suspected Financial Abuse" is required annually for all brokerage employees, whether they deal with customers or not. The training outlines the elements of elder financial abuse, its impact on the victims, and procedures an employee should use to determine when to suspect elder abuse and where to report it.

In addition to this training, in April 2013 WFA launched its first live training for brokerage financial advisors and client associates (FAs and CAs)[10] on elder financial abuse. FAs and CAs are often "first responders" to potential elder financial abuse. This training uses four brief video vignettes to help lead the trainees through group discussions about elder financial abuse scenarios that they might see in their dealings with clients. WFA plans to present this live training to other Wells Fargo FAs and CAs around the country.

Centralized Unit

Essential to a financial services' company's ability to address the epidemic of elder financial abuse is the creation of a centralized response unit. WFA's field personnel are trained to contact their manager and also call a toll-free number for a centralized response unit designed to take reports of potential elder financial abuse. The response unit, which is currently located

---

[10] Financial advisors are the professionals holding one or more licenses permitting them to provide financial services to clients. Client associates are often also licensed and they assist the FAs in servicing their clients.

in the Legal Department of WFA, consists of lawyers and paralegals who do intake, gather clarifying or follow-up information to determine whether the matter is reportable as suspected elder abuse, and then take steps to see that a report is filed with the appropriate APS.[11] While there is a split among the states as to whether financial services firms are "mandatory reporters," Wells Fargo's corporate policy is to consider itself a mandatory reporter of suspected elder and vulnerable adult abuse in all states.

Having a centralized reporting unit for financial abuse offers many advantages. A consistent company response will be given no matter where the report has arisen. In a decentralized model, you may have those making reports in one state apply a completely different, and possibly contrary, method of handling cases from those in other states, even though the cases are similar. Another advantage of centralization is the inherent increase in the expertise level as the team members handle more cases and can share circumstances and nuances with each other. Centralization also allows the unit to work in an advisory role where situations occur that may not be reportable elder financial abuse matters, but where the FAs and CAs can benefit from a discussion of some possible resources. The response unit members have quarterly meetings with others at WFA who touch on some of the elder abuse issues (e.g., fraud investigators and regulatory lawyers) to discuss external challenges and case histories. Finally, the response unit has aided WFA in its effort to gather more data about the number and characteristics of cases of elder financial abuse arising in its nationwide brokerage network (see Figure II-1 for the number of cases coming into the centralized unit in the past year). This information hopefully will allow us to recognize new scam strategies at an earlier time and to refine our client education and FA/CA training on this topic.

Client-Focused Information

Properly designed and distributed information on elder issues can serve the role of a "vaccination" of older individuals against elder financial abuse. It is important that the information is clear, easy to understand, and delivered in a fashion that is balanced and not self-promoting. WFA makes available to the public a comprehensive brochure, *Guide to Financial Protection for the Older Investor*, which covers key topics such as suitable investments, misleading "senior" designations, and instructions on how to identify and report scams. With the assistance of the U.S. Administration on

---

[11] We will use "APS" to refer to state or local agencies that have a statutory obligation to assist older and vulnerable adults in some way. The appropriate name for these agencies and their mission will vary by state. This paper will nonetheless use APS to refer generally to all such agencies.

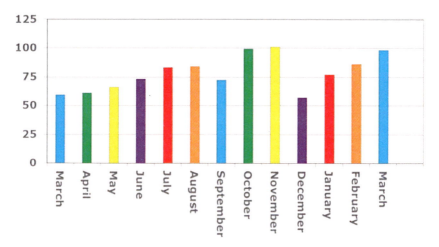

FIGURE II-1 Total elder matters opened March 2012-March 2013.
SOURCE: Wells Fargo Advisors, 2013.

Aging (AoA), WFA recently has started distributing to the public through its FAs and CAs a quick reference guide on elder financial abuse. The pocket-sized brochure describes signs, behaviors, and actions that may be early warnings of financial abuse or exploitation of an older individual. By asking people to speak up and not remain silent, this information will both help prevent potential abuse and increase the likelihood of earlier reporting of an abusive situation. In late spring 2013, Wells Fargo piloted an elder financial abuse awareness program targeting its client base and the public. The seminar provided an interactive forum where the public viewed a summary of a documentary on the challenges of elder financial abuse and then engaged in a discussion with others in the audience as well as experts in the field. WFA believes these client-focused outreach efforts permit financial services companies to work collaboratively with public agencies and other organizations within the community to protect the assets of older people from predators. WFA is evaluating the program for expansion to more locations in the country.

Educational Outreach

WFA is a retail brokerage operation staffed with skilled team members at all levels. With stark self-examination, however, it concluded that it was not as thoroughly educated on the field of elder financial abuse. Accordingly, WFA has taken affirmative steps to increase its knowledge and familiarity with the subject matter. For the past few years, WFA has had a consulting arrangement with Michael Creedon, a well-recognized gerontologist. Creedon has brought his knowledge and expertise to the attention of numerous departments throughout WFA, covering multiple subjects related to elder financial abuse and other issues impacting older Americans.

WFA also sought to learn more about the subject of elder financial abuse by hosting eight half-day symposiums around the country. Joined by professionals from APS, securities regulators, law enforcement, academics, federal agencies, prosecutors, Alzheimer's advocates, medical professions, and other financial services firms, WFA and the participants discussed some challenges facing those detecting and reporting elder financial abuse, particularly in the retail brokerage environment. Using short vignettes to reenact some of the scenarios that financial services firms face, attendees learned, in some instances for the first time, about the structural or attitudinal impediments that actually worked against the seamless and coordinated approach needed to investigate and remediate a case of elder financial abuse. For example, in one symposium, WFA learned that occasionally law enforcement could label a case of potential abuse a "civil matter," and accordingly decline to act. In another instance, WFA learned that what would otherwise seem to be a perfectly well-supported referral to APS could be declined because there was no abuse of government funds or physical injury to the elder victim. While many participants commented after a symposium about how much they benefited from the interactions, the eight gatherings around the country served as an intense "cram" session for WFA as it gathered more insight into the challenges facing the various components of the infrastructure designed to combat elder financial abuse. Indeed, the variations in legislation and in regulations among states, along with the substantial differences around the nation in funding for APS and other response agencies, contribute to the complexity of this issue for multistate financial institutions.

The WFA educational outreach continues by sending staff to conferences and meetings where APS, mental health, and other social service entities often converge to share information and experiences. In 2012, WFA spoke on elder financial abuse at the Oregon Home Care Association's annual conference. Since early 2012, WFA has begun to pair our visits to our state securities regulators with visits to the leadership of that same state's APS agencies. WFA also participated in and presented at the National Adult Protective Services Association's annual conference. At this conference, WFA had opportunities to listen to presentations from a number of APS professionals from around North America. WFA was invited to present at the 19th Annual New York State Abuse Training Institute, whose theme was *Broken Trust: How to Recognize and Respond to Financial Exploitation*. For financial institutions, it will be essential that they continuously educate themselves about elder and vulnerable adults and their susceptibility to various forms of financial abuse. Likewise, financial institutions can contribute their expertise to the education of APS employees, police, and other public-sector professionals who respond to the many ways in which financial abuse can take place.

Partnerships

A final component of a financial institution's inventory of tools to combat elder financial abuse should include a structured use of outside partnerships to help support those who may have a role in stemming the tide of elder financial abuse. As a corporate entity, Wells Fargo has traditionally donated to a number of charitable organizations which in whole or part provided assistance to those who have experienced elder financial or other abuse. Starting in 2012, the firm has embarked on a more focused partnership effort. WFA has joined with other financial services firms to participate in SAFE Team (Security for the Aged from Financial Exploitation Team), a group based in New York City focused on combating elder abuse through identifying and developing best practices for law enforcement, APS, financial institutions, and social services. The AoA has begun working with financial services companies and industry groups to promote programs and educational outreach to raise awareness. While the ink is not dry, Wells Fargo likely will help fund initiatives with some national nonprofits designed to increase training for APS workers on financial and other social service issues as well as training workers and volunteers to carry the prevention of elder abuse message to more seniors and others in communities throughout the country. Though clearly some partnerships are accompanied by an outflow of funds and resources from Wells Fargo, much more is returned to the firm as WFA gains a better and more detailed knowledge of the difficulties inherent in our nation's existing infrastructure designed to handle the rapidly growing elder financial abuse case load.

Top Types of Financial Abuse

The types of financial abuse that affect financial services clients most often fall into the following broad and sometimes overlapping areas of (1) power of attorney (POA) abuse, family disputes, and caregivers; and (2) third-party scams (investments and sweepstakes).

POA Abuse, Family Disputes, and Caregivers

Older clients often use POA documents to give family members and "trusted others" the authority to help them with their financial affairs, partly as a convenience, and also partly in case the older person is suddenly hospitalized, or has another emergency health situation, which may be temporary or permanent. The person who receives that power is referred to as an agent or sometimes an "attorney in fact." The agent has fiduciary duties to the "principal" who granted the power. The agent might be an adult child of the client, a sibling, a caregiver, or a neighbor. When an elder becomes the focus of a dispute between adult children or other family members, over who will "assist" Dad (and Dad's IRA or Dad's bank accounts), it is difficult for a financial services company to figure out whether there are "good guys" or "bad guys." Is this the time to make a report to APS, or do the family members all have Dad's best interests at heart? If the broker is unable to reach the client on the phone to verify that he or she actually has signed a new POA putting her new caregiver on the account, and the caregiver is standing right in front of the broker with instructions to transfer a large sum of money to a new joint bank account, which the caregiver says is needed to pay the client's moving expenses to an assisted living facility—how long should the broker delay that transaction?

The agent whom the older person has chosen is ideally a trusted other who understands that he has a fiduciary duty, and who uses the POA solely for the benefit of the older person. But the agent could also be a thief, who obtained the POA by threats or undue influence, or who sees the powers he has under the POA as a means to accelerate his or her inheritance. Due to recent state laws that were intended to encourage financial institutions to more readily accept POAs (by setting strict time periods, and limiting the reasons to reject a POA, with damages for violations of the law), financial institutions may accept POAs or allow transactions by agents that they would have once rejected as suspicious.

Third-Party Scams (Investments and Sweepstakes)

It is difficult to understand someone who falls victim to a third-party scam, such as the older person from the United States who cannot be shaken from the belief that he or she has won the Malaysian Lottery. Older people who are seemingly capable in every other way have become bitten with the sweepstakes bug, and nothing that law enforcement or the fraud prevention managers of a bank or brokerage tells them can counteract the poison that will cause the older person to deplete all of his or her retirement savings. This depletion occurs often despite protection measures such as giving them newspaper articles or Federal Trade Commission flyers about these scams. With no help from often-overwhelmed law enforcement, no protective services from APS because the client rejects the help, and no cease-and-desist orders from state regulators, it is difficult to impossible for banks and brokerage companies to keep the scammers away from these vulnerable elders.

OWN IT

It appears that mnemonics, acronyms, and catch phrases are often useful in helping drive home the elder financial abuse awareness message. SAFE in New York City and FAST (Financial Abuse Specialists Team) in Houston and other cities are potentially headline-grabbing acronyms that gain needed attention when trying to promote work done by multidisciplinary teams. To this end, WFA has started asking that individuals OWN IT when combating elder abuse. This messaging is summarized below:

Observe: Are there physical changes? Are patterns and habits different? Does the elder behave strangely? Is there a third party present with the elder whose behavior is odd?

Wonder Why: Why is this withdrawal multiples larger than before? Why has the elder just begun to send money to a foreign country?

Negotiate: Can the requested transaction be delayed? Can the check go in two names, elder and trusted third party? Can we only give a fraction of the money today, and more later?

Isolate: Get the elder alone, away from the suspected abuser—"Ms. Smith, please step into my office to confirm some account information," or "Please come with me to discuss some confidential information."

Tattle: Bring your concerns to a supervisor or manager immediately. Use your firm's APS reporting process.

Conclusion

Financial services firms increasingly are playing a greater role in the universal and ongoing struggle to end elder financial abuse. Recounting the efforts of Wells Fargo provides some insight for traditional elder abuse professionals into the various tools and activities that the financial services industry has used. Ideally, this presentation will heighten the awareness of the attendees at the conference regarding challenges faced by these financial firms. In addition, this review may stimulate ideas and discussions on areas of greater collaboration among the financial services industry, the public service agencies that deal with elder abuse issues, and other community organizations that serve elders and their families. We must work together to support our elders and to enable them to have lives of dignity and freedom from abuse.

II.6

ELDER ABUSE AND ITS PREVENTION: SCREENING AND DETECTION

Tara McMullen, M.P.H., Ph.D.(c), and Kimberly Schwartz
Centers for Medicare & Medicaid Services

Mark Yaffe, M.D., C.M., MClSc, CCFP, FCFP
Department of Family Medicine, The McGill University

Scott Beach, Ph.D.
University Center for Social and Urban Research,
University of Pittsburgh

This article reviews information and data presented at the IOM Forum on Global Violence Prevention Workshop on Elder Abuse and Its Prevention. This paper details the screening and detection of elder maltreatment with a focus on the Elder Abuse Suspicion Index (EASI ©). The paper also discusses the measurement of maltreatment within the Physician Quality Reporting System (PQRS) by the Centers for Medicare & Medicaid Services (CMS), and concludes with a more general discussion of issues and challenges in elder abuse screening and detection.

Introduction

The association of elder maltreatment with hospitalizations, hospital admissions, and mortality emphasizes the need to explore and expand appropriate measurement and assessment of maltreatment—across multiple settings and provider types (Mosqueda and Dong, 2011; Dong et al., 2011d, 2012d; Dong, 2012). CMS, among various agencies and stakeholder groups, intends to increase detailed reporting of measures that address a population which warrants representation related to actions of abuse, whether it is neglect, financial, physical, psychological, and/or emotional abuse. Current CMS reporting of maltreatment includes reporting of the *Elder Maltreatment Screen and Follow-up Plan* measure, created for the PQRS, a physician reporting program within CMS. This measure specifically assesses the percentage of patients ages 65 and older with a documented elder maltreatment screen and follow-up plan on the date of positive screen (CMS, 2013). This measure has been reported since 2009 in each reporting period for patients seen by the provider.

Following the inception of the *Elder Maltreatment Screen and Follow-up Plan* measure into the PQRS program, CMS has intended to expand the measurement of elder maltreatment to address a larger venue of providers and settings. This is based on the understanding that opportunities to screen for elder abuse are not just confined to the physician's office or emergency department (McMullen and Schwartz, 2012). Moreover, CMS would like to encourage greater participation in the reporting of elder maltreatment (McMullen and Schwartz, 2012). As noted from preliminary statistics of the *Elder Maltreatment Screen and Follow-up Plan* (2012) measure, the incidence of applicable denominator cases reported in the first 6 months of 2012 were 53,915,669. That is, nearly 54 million individuals were eligible to receive a maltreatment screen when visiting their physician. Of these 54 million reported cases, only 1,438 individuals were actually screened for maltreatment. Cases were reported by psychologists, geriatricians, and occupational therapists, among others. This number reflects the very low participation in reporting of this measure by eligible providers, addressing the need to encourage reporting of elder abuse from a patient safety perspective and patient engagement, and, quite possibly, the expansion of this measure (Quality Insights Pennsylvania, 2013).

The CMS *Elder Maltreatment and Care Symposium*

With a defined focus on expanded reporting and assessment of elder maltreatment, CMS hosted the *Elder Maltreatment and Care Symposium* to explore the current state of elder maltreatment screening and elder care practices across Medicare and Medicaid beneficiary populations and care settings. Moreover, this symposium attempted to develop a framework to build a more comprehensive measure specification for the PQRS. Preliminary analyses from this symposium suggest:

1. There is a consensus that there should be consistency in how to define elder maltreatment across HHS agencies;
2. Crosscutting screening tools are available and could be used in various care settings, by multiple providers, and may evaluate elder abuse and burden on the provider. Three screening tools were identified for increased use in practice for the screening of elder maltreatment (EASI, HS-EAST, and the Vulnerability to Abuse Screening Scale, or VASS). These tools were identified for their ability to assess multiple types of abuse, for the specifications of the measure, and for the focus of each tool when combined;
3. The impact of screening on the provider–patient relationship should be taken into account;
4. Cultural diversity should always be considered in any elder maltreatment measurement; and
5. Awareness of the feasibility and burden on the provider should be kept in mind.

Many questions continue to exist within the domain of elder maltreatment measurement and assessment. Detection, assessment, and reporting of abuse from multiple providers in different settings are imperative. With a focus on assessments, there are uncertainties about what factors are most important to screen for, and what the most valid, reliable assessment tools are. In collaboration with the IOM and CMS, Dr. Mark Yaffe and Dr. Scott Beach discussed factors for screening maltreatment, detailing specifications of a reliable and valid tool for assessment of maltreatment: EASI.

The Elder Abuse Suspicion Index

EASI was conceptualized and validated to respond to the following realities: (1) family physicians are well positioned to try to identify elder abuse, and therefore a tool was necessary for use in the ambulatory office setting; (2) to promote compliance by family physicians with tool usage, the time to administer it needed to be very short, while using language content that was acceptable to them; (3) research ethics requirements would limit validation to those aged 65 or older with Folstein MMSE (Mini-Mental State Examination) scores of 24 or greater; and (4) a tool meeting these requirements would be useful for screening or case finding, but given the complexity of elder abuse, the minimum expectation of the tool would be to generate suspicion about the presence of mistreatment or neglect sufficient to justify further discussion of the issue between doctor and patient, or patient referral to a community expert in elder abuse for in-depth evaluation (Yaffe et al., 2008).

The validated EASI consists of six questions, five asked by the doctor to older adults, and one answered by the doctor based on observation of the patients. Of the doctors in the validation study, in responding to a post-tool usage survey, 96 percent indicated the tool was somewhat to very easy to use, two-thirds doing so in 2 minutes or less. In collaboration with the World Health Organization (WHO), EASI has been shown to have content validity in seven diverse countries (WHO, 2013). There are eight known linguistic versions of the EASI—English, French, German, Hebrew, Italian, Japanese, Portuguese, and Spanish (Yaffe et al., 2012).

Self-administration of the EASI in a slightly modified form (EASI-sa) has been shown to be feasible, acceptable, and comprehensible. This approach also appears to improve seniors' awareness of elder abuse and its manifestations (Yaffe et al., 2012).

In Canada, through a collaboration of the EASI team and the National Initiative for the Care of the Elderly, the EASI has been distributed as a pocket card to 24,000 primary care doctors; there is also a digital version of the tool available online. To date, however, there are no data on the actual uptake of the tool.

Because professionals from various disciplines may approach elder abuse differently, it is productive to explore use of the EASI by different groups (Yaffe et al., 2009). For example, the validation of the EASI in Spain was accomplished using social workers (Perez-Rojo et al., 2010). Meanwhile, in Canada there are preliminary attempts by others in Canada to study nurses' use of EASI in emergency rooms and nursing home settings. No data have been published yet on these two experiences.

Elder Abuse Screening and Detection

Both the CMS work and that of Dr. Yaffe and his colleagues on the EASI focus primarily on screening for elder abuse in health care settings. This last section provides a broad, though necessarily brief, summary and overview of elder abuse screening and detection. The section is summarized in Table II-1. Note that references cited in the text below are examples and not meant to be comprehensive.

Screening and Detection in Community-Dwelling Older Adults

As shown in the table, a variety of approaches have been used to attempt to screen for and detect elder abuse in community-dwelling older adults. One of the key challenges facing the elder abuse field is developing methods for detection in cognitively impaired older adults. As shown, direct victim surveys of both general and disease-specific populations are possible for cognitively intact persons (Laumann et al., 2008; Acierno et al., 2010), but not for those who are cognitively impaired. For impaired populations, researchers must use more indirect methods such as caregiver or potential perpetrator surveys (Wiglesworth et al., 2010), health care provider screening, reports from social service providers or others who come into frequent contact with older adults ("sentinels") (National Center on Elder Abuse, 1998), and forensic analysis of bruising patterns (Wiglesworth et al., 2009). Note that all of these techniques are also appropriate for cognitively intact older adults. Of course, official APS reports can also be used, but there is general agreement that elder abuse is greatly underreported and that these official reports represent merely the "tip of the iceberg" (NRC, 2003).

Screening and Detection in Institutionalized Older Adults

Paralleling community-dwelling methods, long-term care resident surveys are also possible for those who are cognitively intact, although these direct surveys are somewhat rare. More common methods applicable to both cognitively intact and cognitively impaired residents—who make up

TABLE II-1 Overview Summary of Elder Abuse Screening and Detection Methods and General Issues/Challenges

Methods for Community-Dwelling Older Adults	Methods for Institutionalized Older Adults
• Direct victim surveys (random sample)* • Direct victim surveys (targeted disease)* • Direct caregiver surveys (targeted disease) • Direct perpetrator surveys • Health care screening (physicians, emergency department, hospital, dental clinics) • Community "sentinels" • Social service providers (adult day care) • Forensic analysis (bruising) • APS/official reports	• Resident surveys* • Staff surveys • Family surveys • Resident informant/proxy surveys • Forensic analysis (bruising) • Video monitoring of public areas • Long-term care (LTC) ombudsman/official reports (Both staff–resident and resident–resident abuse)

General Issues and Challenges

- Elder abuse from whose perspective? Older adult victims? Clinicians? Proxy informants?
- If cognitively intact, should we always get the victim's perspective? (maintain autonomy versus "objectivity" of clinicians?)
- General self-report issues (accuracy, disclosure, motivation, etc.)
- Health care provider compliance with screening
- Access to and cooperation from long-term care facilities
- Which screening/measurement tool to use? (many options may need more psychometric testing, development)
- Interviews vs. self-administered? Technology for data collection? (impact on perceived privacy, comfort reporting)
- Setting, context important—own home, primary care physician's office, waiting room, emergency department (impact on perceived privacy, comfort reporting)
- Neglect particularly challenging—omission (not helping) or commission (actively preventing access to food, water, medicine)? Co-occurrence with self-neglect?
- Financial exploitation also especially challenging—stranger fraud/scams versus family/trusted others (different dynamics)
- Sensitivity to the wider cultural context

* Cognitively intact only.

a large portion of the institutionalized population—include staff surveys (Castle and Beach, 2013) and family member surveys (Zhang et al., 2012). These methods have been used to detect both staff-to-resident and resident-to-resident abuse, which Lachs and colleagues (2007) have argued are the most prevalent forms of abuse occurring in long-term care settings.

Resident informant/proxy surveys are also a possibility, as is forensic bruising analyses (Wiglesworth et al., 2009). An intriguing though unexplored possibility is the use of video monitoring and direct observation of staff–resident and resident–resident interaction in public areas such as hallways and dining areas. Finally, official ombudsman reports are also available, but likely represent only a small portion of the cases actually occurring.

General Issues and Challenges in Elder Abuse Screening and Detection

The methods briefly reviewed above each have both strengths and weaknesses. Elder abuse is a largely hidden phenomenon that people are reluctant to acknowledge, much less discuss openly with strangers. Table II-1 summarizes a few of the key issues and challenges that confront researchers and health care providers as they attempt to screen for and detect elder abuse. They include issues around autonomy versus clinician "objectivity," potential self-report issues, health care provider compliance, access to and cooperation from long-term care facilities, selection of appropriate tools and measures, mode of data collection and use of technology, and how the setting or context in which the abuse screening or questioning occurs may affect responses. As one example, Dr. Scott Beach's work has shown that removing the interviewer from the situation in direct victim surveys through use of survey technologies like audio computer-assisted self-interviewing (A-CASI) can result in prevalence rates for financial and psychological abuse that are two to three times higher than when an interviewer asks the questions (Beach et al., 2010). In contrast, older adults may be more willing to tell their physician directly about abuse given increased trust and rapport. As screening for elder abuse in health care settings becomes more common through the previously described work of CMS, issues around health care provider compliance and the best tools and methods for different care settings (physician offices, emergency department, dental clinics, etc.) will need to be addressed. Table II-1 also notes that neglect and financial exploitation pose unique challenges for screening and detection. Finally, any effort to screen for and detect elder abuse must be sensitive to the wider cultural context, and interesting work is occurring both among diverse groups in the United States (Dong and Simon, 2010; DeLiema, 2012) and in the international context (WHO, 2008).

II.7

ELDER ABUSE AND NEGLECT: A ROLE FOR PHYSICIANS

James G. O'Brien, M.D.
University of Louisville, Kentucky

Elder abuse continues to be neglected as a problem that adversely affects older adults, robbing them of quality of life and, on occasion, resulting in death. Self-neglect is the orphan in the spectrum of abuse and neglect; it is perhaps the most challenging to deal with, and in some states is excluded from definitions of abuse and neglect.

Until recently, physicians appeared to play a very minor role in detection and reporting of cases of elder abuse, in contrast with child abuse, where pediatricians had and continue to have a major role in detection, intervention, research, reporting, and development of creative model programs for combating the problem. In addition, they have been instrumental in launching a massive public health initiative to acquaint the public with the problem. By contrast, elder abuse and neglect receives a fraction of the funding from states and remains chronically underfunded in the area of research.

Physicians are perceived to contribute very little as judged by frequency of reporting, but this may not accurately reflect the contribution of physicians. Some recent studies of elder abuse and neglect in Ireland have identified physicians as being eighth in rank of reporting (Clancy et al., 2011). Yet, a study of general practitioners revealed significant involvement in terms of identification and intervention.

A survey of general practitioners in Ireland in 2010 revealed nearly two-thirds had encountered cases, with 35.5 percent encountering a case in the past year (O'Brien et al., 2013a). Most cases were detected by the general practitioners during a home visit. In addition, 13.3 percent had been threatened by a perpetrator or family member. Nearly three-quarters, 73 percent, perceived their role to becoming involved beyond medical care. Finally, 70 percent of general practitioners believed the situation for the victim had improved after intervention.

A survey of geriatricians in Ireland and Scotland in 2010 regarding self-neglect revealed most had encountered cases in the past year, with personal neglect and refusal of services being common presentations. Interestingly, 40 percent of cases were thought to contain elements of abuse, which is not surprising given the vulnerability of the individuals. Dementia, lifelong personality traits, depression, and alcoholism were cited as the most common underlying causes. Comprehensive geriatric evaluation was identified as the most appropriate intervention. The respondents identified the need for more education for geriatricians and others in health care (Bartley et al., 2011).

A survey of psychiatrists specializing in care for elderly patients in Ireland in 2010 regarding self-neglect revealed significant exposure, with 92 percent having seen a case in the past year. Personal characteristics, loss of self-care, and poor hygiene were the most common presentations. Medication non-compliance and hoarding were the next most common. In contrast with the geriatricians, 59 percent believed the outcome for the patient was unsatisfactory. Nearly three-quarters, 72 percent, believed the outcome for themselves as psychiatrists was unsatisfactory (O'Brien et al., 2013b).

Apparently, at least in Ireland, using reports from physicians as an indication of involvement in abuse and neglect may seriously underestimate their contributions. Perhaps the same applies in the United States and other countries.

Another area of unrecognized abuse occurs within the health care system with multiple examples of overtreatment (not indicated/futile) constituting abuse. The corollary occurs when indicated treatments are withheld because of age, resulting in neglect. These situations rarely come to the attention of any agency and stay below the radar. This is an area that urgently requires more investigation.

II.8

PREVENTING ELDER ABUSE—HOPE SPRINGS ETERNAL

Elizabeth Podnieks, C.M., Ed.D.
Ryerson University, Founder of World Elder Abuse Awareness Day

Cynthia Thomas, Ph.D.
Westat

Introduction

The abuse of older people is a global issue that has been receiving increased attention as the aging population grows. Although progress has been made, there is still a lack of scientific research, and limited policies and tools for interventions. This paper reflects on some perspectives from the field since the publication of the landmark study by Dr. Alexandre Kalache (WHO, 2002), *Missing Voices*. That study, for the first time, actually asked older people to tell their stories, recorded and published them, and invited the elder abuse community to build on these stories and seek ways to incorporate them into interventions and practice initiatives. One of the strongest, most poignant comments—"respect is better than food and water"—resonates through the concepts discussed here: elder abuse prevention networks, support groups, global awareness, engaging youth, social media, and the need for an elder abuse conceptual framework.

Networks: Demonstrated Leadership

The 1980s and 1990s saw the emergence of networks for the prevention of elder abuse. They began as small grassroots initiatives that brought together people who were concerned with the growing reports about elder abuse and neglect both in the community and in long-term care facilities. Members included researchers, educators, practitioners, and advocates dedicated to protecting the safety, security, and dignity of older persons. The organizers were passionate visionaries who developed effective ways of providing support to individuals and families caught in abusive situations. The networks lobbied the government and set up hotlines with volunteers. It was not unusual for a victim to call a network member at 1 AM with the question, "Can't the police just get my money back?" Meeting minutes were kept in a filing cabinet at a university and meetings were held in empty classrooms. The police were among the most generous network members and would bring supplies for workshops and provide transportation, much to the appreciation of the people who were being helped. Today, networks have been established in most developed countries; there are funding, offices, and available resources. The initial goals remain strong; networks are a force for connection, communication, and sharing. They seek to achieve a clearer understanding of elder abuse and provide leadership to prevent it.

Networks have assumed an important role in identifying and supporting regional, national, and local activities related to World Elder Abuse Awareness Day (WEAAD) and in providing links to the international scene. The planning for this annual event has indeed become a core event of many networks. Today, networks serve to promote elder abuse prevention through education, professional training, advocacy, and service coordination, and in so doing, bring the safety, protection, and respect that was called for in *Missing Voices*.

Support Groups: A Chance for Human Connection

Support groups have been helpful to victims of elder abuse (Podnieks, 1999). The early networks organized support groups because they were inexpensive and accessible, and they filled a huge need in the lives of victims by providing guidance in handling difficult situations. Support groups are able to relieve the tensions, resentments, and stress that accompany elder abuse. They also provide a safe and caring environment as victims navigate the health, legal, and social systems and address their own needs and concerns. Support groups provide a safe environment, allowing victims to ask questions such as, "Why does my son abuse me?" Counseling should be offered to those who need it. The groups encourage members to express their feelings of anger, frustration, guilt, resentment, and hopelessness, and assist participants in asserting more control in their own situations (Kaasaslainen, 2000). Support group members often can heal, find resolution, and return as volunteer support group facilitators.

Support groups for caregivers promote an opportunity to discuss circumstances that may lead to mistreatment, such as stress, anger, feelings of entrapment, anxiety, sense of disruption in life, and role changes (Podnieks, 1999). The informal nature of the group establishes a setting for free and safe conversations about situations that abused older persons, caregivers, and staff in long-term facilities had not been able to discuss with others. Support groups encourage people to speak of the unthinkable, to bolster each other, and to help solve each other's problems.

World Elder Abuse Awareness Day

Clearly one of the most significant accomplishments of network collaboration was the launching of WEAAD on June 15, 2006. The goal was to build momentum at international, regional, and national levels to raise awareness of elder abuse and the need to prevent it. WEAAD has heightened global consciousness and strengthened leadership networks: It has been a compelling force on human rights, aging, and the prevention of family violence. The concept of World Day was spread across all nations, absorbing influences from other traditions. What began as a small gathering at the United Nations in 2006 has evolved into a multicultural, multilingual movement that is redefining the meaning of collective power for a world audience. WEAAD has helped people understand what elder abuse is, the importance of human and civil rights, and the need for research, education, advocacy, and policy development. In 2011, the United Nations officially designated June 15 as WEAAD, an idea that has been embraced by nongovernmental organizations, government agencies, health and social care providers, law enforcement professionals, aging advocates, and many others. In a historic moment on June 15, 2012, President Obama held a workshop on elder abuse at the White House and issued a Presidential Proclamation.

Power of Youth

Children and youth are an untapped resource for preventing elder abuse; they are society's most engaging and powerful change agents. If they are taught about elder abuse and given the opportunity to become engaged in community-based work with older adults, they can help to prevent it.

Education about elder abuse begins with instilling positive images of aging and older persons in children, beginning with preschool so that it becomes a way of thinking that grows through life. Elder abuse awareness education should continue throughout secondary school and higher. Elder abuse advocates recognize the importance of changing ageist attitudes in both young and older generations. The good news is that most children are willing to help to raise awareness in their community if they are asked and included in the planning. Some examples of student participation include developing posters and slogans, visiting nursing homes, handing out pamphlets, speaking to banks, working with the police, and participating in social media. When students learn about elder abuse at school, they can take the information home to their parents. Young people often have strong ties to their grandparents, and these feelings must be nurtured. Findings from the World View Environmental Scan (Podnieks et al., 2010) indicated that older people desperately want to be connected to the world of technology. The lack of resources to foster these connections is a gap that needs to be addressed. Young people can help, and benefit in return. One such example is that of a teen teaching an elder how to use the computer while she helped him with his math homework, showing reciprocity in action, or exchange theory.

Projects both in schools and in the community are being developed to make young people aware of and sensitive to old age. In so doing, it is hoped that children and young people will develop greater respect for the elderly and will be much less inclined, now and in the future, to mistreat them. Schools also are including the topic of conflict resolution in their curriculums, and teachers have found that a discussion of elder abuse can be introduced as part of this topic (Podnieks, 2002).

Changing the World, One Click at a Time

The social media offers unique opportunities to engage a worldwide audience in the challenge of addressing elder abuse and neglect. Through global communication we can reach people and places that have been unable to access tools, resources, and network meetings. Cyberspace has become a resource for ongoing elder abuse prevention strategies. The possibilities for knowledge transfer through virtual learning are exciting and far reaching. Cyberspace promises to create an expansive Internet platform reaching millions of people. In using all the tools of social media, a groundswell can be generated that will lead to a greater sense of community, of citizenship, and of human connection. A challenge is to ensure that older people, who have been left out of the technological revolution, can use the Internet and have the opportunity to access information that greatly affects them.

Another area of global technology applicable to elder abuse awareness and prevention is Geo Mapping. Online mapping and information tools can facilitate opportunities for people from a wide geographic area to share information. Members of the community can share strategies in multiple settings. The tool can allow successful projects, research, and policies to be shared through an online forum. The Geo Map can visually show the location of elder abuse networks, organizations, and individuals throughout the world, as well as their activities, projects, and resources. The map can be a powerful visual tool to display for government and others the potential locations of leadership (McKee, 2010).

Generating a Conceptual Framework

For many years, scholars, researchers, practitioners, policy makers, and others have been calling for a conceptual framework that is specific to elder abuse and neglect. Elder abuse has been referred to as "a-theoretical," borrowing from theoretical models from sociology, psychology, feminism, health promotion, and the fields of child abuse and domestic violence (Podnieks, 2002). Tremendous strides have been made in the field, and now is an opportune time to develop a framework that will consolidate these elements from useful theories that have been guiding elder abuse work.

It is difficult to work without a common frame of reference in addressing and understanding the complexity of elder abuse and neglect. Existing theories have not been tested and evaluated within the context of elder abuse. A theory must be developed that includes the characteristics of both victims and their abusers—their cognitive statuses, the nature of their relationships, the types of abuse, settings, and protective factors (Jackson and Hafemeister, 2013). It is important to examine existing models as we search for our own theory. For example, elder abuse can be considered a health care issue. The Determinants of Health model proposed by WHO offers valuable insights into factors that impact elder abuse. Other factors may be relevant to theory development, such as caregiver stress or dependency. Ageism may be a factor (McDonald, 2011).

Exchange theory suggests that abuse can result through dependency and reciprocity between the abused and the abuser. Social learning theory refers to behaviors learned in childhood that are repeated in adulthood. The ecological model sees abuse as the result of the complex interplay among a person's individual characteristics, the community, and social factors. The lifecourse approach links the individual and the social structure to accumulative advantage/disadvantage over time (McDonald, 2013). Missing from many theories but critical to a new elder abuse theory is a human rights approach, which will frame social justice and health equity and reinforce the civil and human rights of all people. The restorative justice approach has been used with some success in Canada. Researchers continue to debate on conceptual frameworks. At a recent workshop, a participant stated, "we don't use a model . . . we prefer to go out and just do it." That approach may work in some situations, but the time has come for those in the elder abuse prevention field to articulate a solid conceptual framework. How can we teach students and beginning practitioners without a road map and without guidelines?

This paper calls for the formation of a global work party to generate a conceptual framework that belongs to and reflects the philosophy of elder abuse. It has been talked about by many scholars, researchers, and practitioners—it is an idea whose time has come, and the commitment and passion are there to accomplish it. A call has gone out to the international community; an action plan will be generated and the concept will become a work in progress. Garrison (2000, p. 3) best articulates why elder abuse researchers must now generate a framework for elder abuse: "Theoretical inquiry is central to the vitality and development of a field of practice—not to mention its recognition and credibility from those not yet initiated into the field. The theoretical foundations of a field describe and inform the practice and provide the primary means to guide future developments. It influences practices and research, reveals new knowledge and suggests alternatives."

Summary

Elder abuse is a universal problem. Research shows that it is prevalent in both the developed and developing world. Enhancing understanding and raising awareness is the responsibility of all countries, and the more that can be shared the more effective the outcomes. The strategies described in this paper can be applied at a global level. The use of social media makes it possible to communicate around the world and to be connected with programs and practice in many countries.

This paper has been a brief reflection of the historical field of elder abuse and some milestones: the evolution of networks and support groups, initiatives such as WEAAD, and the emergence of the role of technology. This paper closes with a call and a vision for the theorists of the field to describe what we have learned and map what we know in order to discover what is not known.

II.9

ELDER ABUSE INTERVENTION: THE SHELTER MODEL AND THE LONG-TERM CARE FACILITY

Daniel A. Reingold, J.D., M.S.W., Joy Solomon, Esq., and Malya Levin, Esq.
The Weinberg Center for Elder Abuse Prevention and Research, The Hebrew Home at Riverdale

"We are not here to curse the darkness, but to light the candle that can guide us through that darkness to a safe and sane future."

—John F. Kennedy, Presidential Nomination Acceptance Speech

In 2004, when the Harry and Jeanette Weinberg Center for Elder Abuse Prevention at The Hebrew Home at Riverdale, New York, the nation's first regional elder abuse shelter, was founded, many of the critical studies regarding the astounding prevalence of elder abuse had not yet been released. The community was not yet aware that there had been a 19.7 percent increase in elder abuse incidents between 2000 and 2004 (Wood, 2006), or that financial exploitation results in a national annual loss to victims of $2.9 billion (MetLife Mature Market Institute, 2011). When Dan Reingold, the CEO of The Hebrew Home at Riverdale, and Joy Solomon, then the director of elder abuse services at the Pace Women's Justice Center, created this new model of intervention for elder abuse victims, they were not aware that for every elder abuse incident documented by government agencies in New York state, there are 23 more that go unreported (Lifespan of Greater Rochester et al., 2011). Instead of investigating the exact nature of the darkness of elder abuse, they decided to "light a candle" by conceiving, planning, and manifesting a unique model of acute elder abuse intervention: a cost-effective, highly adaptable, multifaceted, and easily replicable partnership with a preexisting long-term care facility.

Cost-Effective

Research has shown that, preexisting health issues notwithstanding, a victim of elder abuse is more than twice as likely to use a hospital emergency room than his or her counterpart who has not been the victim of abuse (Dong, 2005). Therefore, any effective prevention method will result in a dramatic lowering of health care costs. The shelter model has the additional and significant advantage of leveraging the extensive preexisting resources of a long-term care community to create a service that provides a high level of care at a low variable cost.

Long-term care facilities already operate with many of the features critical to the success of an elder abuse shelter. They are open 7 days a week. They are nearly guaranteed to have a bed available at all times. They maintain a skilled nursing and therapeutic staff that has undergone mandated elder abuse training. Short-term, emergency placement in a residence with a caring staff and a broad range of activities designed to build community, capacity, and a sense of fulfillment is a critical first step toward healing for Weinberg Center clients.

Highly Adaptable

At its core, an elder abuse shelter just needs a bed to fulfill the essential mission of providing a haven of safety and protection for victims of abuse. Beyond that, victims are integrated into the long-term care facility's preexisting community, whatever form it takes. These victims are placed within the facility as appropriate for their medical needs, and are not publicly identified as participants in the shelter program. At the Weinberg Center, only the shelter's dedicated staff knows exactly who their clients are. All staff must be trained about procedures and guidelines unique to abuse victims. There are special admission procedures, as well as a different attitude toward family involvement. Although family involvement is generally actively encouraged and facilitated at The Hebrew Home, Weinberg Center clients usually consent to a total visitation moratorium for their first 2 weeks of stay at the shelter. The Weinberg Center has found that this buffer zone of adjustment and recuperation has been extremely advantageous to clients' well-being. While a long-term care facility's staff will need to adjust to some of these operational variances, they will largely be able to seamlessly integrate the shelter population into their preexisting functions.

A shelter program also capitalizes on a long-term care facility's community partners, and provides the residence with an opportunity to maximize and expand those connections. APS, often the first responders to incidents of elder abuse, are critical partners in connecting a shelter with its community catchment area. Once the Weinberg Center had basic shelter infrastructure in place, it began to incorporate community outreach and training as a fundamental part of its mission. Weinberg Center staff have conducted educational series on the signs, symptoms, and appropriate responses to elder abuse for a broad gamut of professional and community groups. These groups include hospital and health care employees, law enforcement workers, financial institution employees, legislators, and even door attendants. These cohorts are all positioned to identify and intervene in instances of suspected elder abuse, and to help refer clients to the Weinberg Center where appropriate.

The Hebrew Home has also created a screening process that connects the Weinberg Center with the wide network of services the Home operates across the continuum of care. Every new resident of The Hebrew Home undergoes a screening process designed by Weinberg Center staff with the goal of identifying instances of possible elder abuse. These cases are flagged for further investigation by the Weinberg Center's Community Health Specialist. Through a grant from the Robin Hood Foundation, this program has now been expanded to include clients in The Hebrew Home's short-term rehab facility as well as community residents who are clients of The Hebrew Home's managed long-term care service. Ten thousand older adults are serviced by this network of preexisting programs, which, with relatively slight modifications, has become a part of, and helped to strengthen and enlarge, the Weinberg Center's referral system.

Multifaceted

With time-tested operational practices and robust community partnerships, the Weinberg Center has turned its attention to broader policy issues affecting older adults, with a heavy emphasis on protection and restitution via the civil legal system. The Weinberg Center has three attorneys on staff, and looks for opportunities to pursue victims' rights as well as to advocate for expansions and changes in the law that will further protect and consider those rights.

One such endeavor is a protocol that has been adopted by several of New York City's Family Courts to allow homebound and mobility-challenged older adults to obtain orders of protection without the long and physically demanding process of attending a courtroom proceeding. In the Weinberg Center's experience, a civil order of protection issued against an abuser is a powerful weapon in a shelter's legal arsenal. Typically, a petitioner must first come to court for an initial appearance and the issuance of a temporary order of protection. The petitioner must then arrange for service of process on the alleged abuser. Finally, the victim must return to court on a second date for a hearing and issuance of a final order of protection. The onerous travel and wait times and logistical arrangements required by this process have a significant chilling effect on victims of elder abuse considering this route. Having observed this phenomenon repeatedly, the Weinberg Center's legal staff have been at the forefront of advocating and assisting with implementation of a protocol that allows local community agencies, such as Family Justice Centers, to assist older adult victims in submitting, retrieving, and serving court papers as well as making telephonic court appearances. Currently, courts in the Bronx, Brooklyn, Manhattan, and Queens have implemented this protocol (Lok, 2012). In this way, the Weinberg Center is working to streamline its own civil legal services, as well as to assist the broader community in creating an effective toolkit to combat elder abuse.

As much as the Weinberg Center champions maximal usage of the civil and criminal legal systems, part of its mission includes tackling cutting-edge issues, such as the disturbingly fine line between older adult sexual expression and abuse, where the law still lags behind the current reality. While the right to robust sexual expression as well as the right to live free from abuse are both fundamental to our legal system, it is often difficult to determine the exact nature of a cognitively impaired older adult's sexual activity. The Weinberg Center team and The Hebrew Home's Memory Care Director and Sexual Rights Advocate have partnered to address this sensitive issue via a mixed legal and therapeutic lens, crafting a protocol and an accompanying presentation appropriate for a variety of legal and health care audiences. By collaborating with The Hebrew Home's expert staff, the Weinberg Center strives to expand the reach of both organizations by working toward shared goals.

Easily Replicable

Shortly after the Weinberg Center opened in 2005, the Center began to encourage and support replication of its shelter model in other long-term care facilities. It has successfully assisted in the creation of and/or ongoing development of those replications in more than 10 independent facilities. In the past year, as the movement to create shelters continued to gain momentum, the Weinberg Center created the SPRiNG Alliance (Shelter Partners: Regional, National, Global) to lend structure to its replication program. SPRiNG Alliance's mission is to create a network of regional elder abuse shelters and similar service models with close working relationships, shared resources and technical assistance, common standards of excellence, and a vibrant community of support. The Alliance currently conducts monthly phone calls and maintains a website with shared resources at www.spring-alliance.org, and held its inaugural Symposium in May 2013. The creation of this alliance heralds the groundswell of momentum that has coalesced around the shelter model, and has become a critical part of the Weinberg Center's mission.

Partnership

The relationship between the Weinberg Center and The Hebrew Home is truly symbiotic, helping both entities to leverage their resources, maximize their capacity, and extend their reach. While the structural and operational benefits to the Weinberg Center in partnering with The Hebrew Home have been discussed at length above, it is worth highlighting several concrete ways in which the opposite is true. The Hebrew Home's partnership with the Weinberg Center has afforded the Home the opportunity to expand its network of relationship and alliances, opening new entry points to valuable community partnerships. The partnership has connected The Hebrew Home with a plethora of potential funding streams and has been the source of significant media attention for the Home. Additionally, the onsite presence of the Weinberg Center staff allows The Hebrew Home to continue to innovate regarding other family violence–related issues, including, most recently, the implementation of a workplace domestic violence program that includes mandatory training for all staff members.

Most critically, the partnership between The Hebrew Home and the Weinberg Center supports The Hebrew Home's core value of celebrating older adults as unique individuals deserving of dignity and respect. Nationwide, there are currently nearly 5,000 nonprofit, long-term care facilities with more than 750,000 beds nation-wide (Nursing Home Data Compendium, 2010). The success of the partnership between the Weinberg Center and The Hebrew Home at Riverdale demonstrates that all of those beds might one day be part of the burgeoning shelter movement, serving as beacons of hope in the darkness of the lives of elder abuse victims.

II.10

ELDER ABUSE IN ASIA—AN OVERVIEW

Elsie Yan, Ph.D.
Department of Social Work and Social Administration,
University of Hong Kong

The rate of elder abuse is expected to increase as many Asian countries are aging at an unprecedented pace. In 2012, 11 percent of the population in Asia was 60 years and older. By 2050, this percentage is expected to reach 24 percent (Help Age International, 2013).

A substantial amount of research has accumulated on elder abuse in Asian populations, especially Chinese, Indian, Japanese, Korean, and Singaporean. This paper summarizes prevalence estimates of elder abuse in these populations. Special attention is paid to the reviewing of scholarly works that reflect on the unique culture in Asia relevant to the understanding of elder abuse.

Prevalence of Elder Abuse in Asia

Considerable variation, with rates ranging from 0.22 per 1,000 to 62 percent, has been observed in the prevalence estimates of elder abuse across

Asia. Psychological abuse and neglect are frequently reported in studies using older persons or their caregivers as informants. Physical violence and financial abuse are more commonly observed in cases identified in the clinical setting and in cases reported to governmental or nongovernmental organizations.

People's Republic of China (PRC)

Published work on elder abuse estimates in the PRC mainly came from two studies. In the first study of a convenience sample of 412 older Chinese attending an urban medical center in Nanjing, Dong and his colleagues (Dong et al., 2007a; Dong and Simon, 2008, 2010) reported a prevalence of 35 percent, with caregiver neglect being the most common form of mistreatment (16.9 percent), followed by financial exploitation (13.6 percent), emotional abuse (11.4 percent), physical abuse (5.8 percent), sexual abuse (1.2 percent), and abandonment (0.7 percent). Thirty-six percent of the participants in this sample experienced two or more types of abuse.

The second study involves 2,000 older Chinese recruited through two-stage cluster sampling, in Hubei. Wu and his colleagues (2012) reported similar prevalence rates of 36.2 percent, with psychological abuse being the most common form of mistreatment (27.3 percent), followed by caregiver neglect (15.8 percent), physical abuse (4.9 percent), and financial exploitation (2 percent). Ten percent of the participants in this study suffered multiple forms of elder mistreatment.

Hong Kong

Based on a convenience sample of 355 older Chinese, prevalence rates of 2 percent for physical abuse and 20.8 percent for verbal abuse have been reported (Yan and Tang, 2001). Another study of 276 older Chinese indicated that 27.5 percent of the older respondents reported having experienced at least one abusive behavior by their family caregiver during the surveyed year (Yan and Tang, 2004). The most common form of abuse in this sample was verbal abuse (26.8 percent), whereas violation of personal rights (5.1 percent) and physical abuse (2.5 percent) were comparatively rare.

In a sample of 122 family caregivers of older persons with dementia recruited from local community centers, 62 percent and 18 percent of the caregivers reported having verbally or physically abused the care recipients in the past month (Yan and Kwok, 2010). In a study of 464 younger adults, 20 percent, 2.4 percent, and 2.4 percent indicated they would verbally, physically, or socially abuse an older person if there is no social constraint and that no punishment whatsoever would follow (Yan and Tang, 2003).

Taiwan

In Taiwan, 195 older Chinese subjects, both institutionalized and community-dwelling older Chinese, completed the Psychological Elder Abuse Scale (Wang, 2006). Participants in this sample endorsed an average of 6.32 psychologically abusive behaviors. More commonly reported behaviors were: "wishes to see relatives unfulfilled" (62.6 percent), "economic dependence on others" (61 percent), and "being left alone involuntarily" (44.1 percent).

Wang (2005) collected information from 114 caregivers in institution settings on the Caregiver Psychological Elder Abuse Behavior Scale. On a possible range of 20-80, participants' mean score was 31.93, indicating most participants engaged in some abusive behaviors. Indeed, only one participant in this sample reported never demonstrating any abusive behaviors toward a care recipient. "Accusing patient verbally" (mean = 2.18), "ignoring patient's requests" (mean = 2.11), and "insulting patient" (mean = 2.02) were the items of the highest mean scores. A similar study of 92 family caregivers (Wang et al., 2006) found a mean score of 30.45, with "blaming him verbally" (mean = 2.06), "ignoring his request" (mean = 1.96), and "refusing to accept his opinions" (mean = 1.86) being the items of the highest mean scores.

Chinese Immigrants in Canada

Lai (2011) reported a prevalence of 4.5 percent in a random sample of 2,272 older Chinese residing in Canada. Of the respondents, 2.5 percent reported having experienced multiple types of mistreatment. The more common abusive acts included "being scolded" (2.5 percent), "being yelled at" (2.4 percent), "being treated impolitely all the time" (1.5 percent), and "being ridiculed" (1.2 percent).

India

In a survey of 864 older women in Pune city, 47 percent reported that they were abused and 40 percent believed they were neglected by their family (Bambawale, 1997).

Chokkanathan and Lee (2006) found a prevalence rate of 14.1 percent in a sample of 400 community-dwelling older Indians, with chronic verbal abuse being the most common (10.8 percent), followed by financial abuse (5 percent), physical abuse (4.3 percent), and neglect (4.3 percent). Among the abused elderly, nearly half reported they had experienced multiple forms of abuse (Chokkanathan and Lee, 2006).

In a representative household survey of 300 older Indians, Sebastian and Sekher (2011) found that nearly half of the respondents (49 percent) reported that they had experienced abuse or neglect from their family members in the surveyed year. Neglect and verbal abuse (39 percent) were the most common forms of mistreatment, followed by physical abuse (13 percent).

In a large-scale representative study conducted by HelpAge India (2012), 31 percent of the 5,400 respondents had experienced abuse and 24 percent faced abuse on a daily basis. More than half of those who were abused had been enduring the abuse for more than 4 years. Among those who reported abuse, 44 percent identified disrespect as the most common form of abuse, 30 percent identified neglect, and 26 percent identified verbal abuse. Forty-six percent of the respondents in this sample had observed cases of abuse in their surroundings.

Singapore

In Singapore, Cham and Seow (2000) reviewed all cases of non-accidental injuries in older persons presenting to the emergency department of a major hospital. Among the 62,826 older patients received between 1994 and 1997, 17 cases of elder abuse were identified, yielding a prevalence rate of 0.3 percent. Using a similar research method, Phua and colleagues (2008) identified 42 cases in 31,145 patients (0.13 percent) presented to the emergency department over a 12-month period. The 42 cases identified involved physical mistreatment (N = 27), neglect (N = 25), psychological mistreatment (N = 6), financial mistreatment (N = 2), abandonment (N = 1), and self-neglect (N = 1).

Japan

In a sample of 78 older Japanese living in an agricultural village, 17.9 percent reported abuse (Anme et al., 2005). Among those who were abused, the most common type of abuse was psychological abuse (50 percent), followed by neglect (42.8 percent), financial exploitation (35.7 percent), physical abuse (21 percent), inadequate administration of medicine (21 percent), self-neglect (14.3 percent), and sexual abuse (7.1 percent) (Anme, 2004).

Attempts have also been made to investigate caregiver reports of abusive behaviors. In a survey of 412 family caregivers of older Japanese who used the visiting nursing services, 34.9 percent reported having engaged in potentially harmful behavior against the older care recipient in the past year (Sasaki et al., 2007). The most frequently reported behaviors were verbal aggression (16.8 percent) and ignoring (13.6 percent). In another survey of 123 Japanese caregivers of older persons referred to a memory clinic, 15.4 percent reported abuse (Kishimoto et al., 2013). Psychological abuse was reported in all cases, and two cases involved both physical and psychological abuse.

In a representative sample of 4,391 older Japanese, more than half had heard of the term "elder abuse" before, among which 18.1 percent personally knew an elder abuse victim (Tsukada et al., 2001).

Cases reported to social services agencies also allow a glimpse at the patterns of elder abuse in Japan. Reviewing a total of 150 elder abuse cases receiving telephone counseling service, Yamada (1999) concluded that financial abuse (49.8 percent) was the most common form of abuse in this sample, followed by psychological abuse (46 percent), physical abuse (35.3 percent), neglect (21.3 percent), self-neglect (1.3 percent), and sexual abuse (0.7 percent).

Despite the relatively high rates of elder abuse reported in the community, official records of elder abuse cases are relatively low in Japan. Reviewing cases identified by officials in 489 municipalities, Nakanishi and colleagues (2010) found a rate of 0.429 per 1,000 in 2008. Based on the responses from 917 municipalities, Nakanishi and other colleagues (2009) estimated that the rate of new reports of suspected cases over a 6-month period was 0.35 per 1,000 and the rate of substantiated cases was 0.22 per 1,000.

South Korea

Drawing from a representative sample of 15,230 older Koreans residing in Seoul, Oh et al. (2006) reported an overall prevalence rate of 6.3 percent for elder abuse. Prevalence of individual types of abuse were: emotional abuse (4.2 percent), financial abuse (4.1 percent), verbal abuse (3.6 percent), neglect (2.4 percent), and physical abuse (1.9 percent).

Lee and Kolomer (2005) interviewed 481 family caregivers providing care to older Koreans with dementia. They found that 16.4 percent had "often yelled at the care recipients," 7.5 percent had often "confined the care recipients to a room," 4 percent had often "left their care recipients unattended," 2.9 percent had often "not prepare[d] a meal for the care recipient," and 14.9 percent of caregivers had "hit the care recipients." In a sample of 934 older Koreans recovering from stroke, prevalence of elder abuse was 13.5 percent (Kim et al., 2012). Emotional abuse was the most frequently reported (10 percent), followed by financial neglect (3.8 percent), caring neglect (3.3 percent), financial abuse (2.1 percent), and physical abuse (1.9 percent).

Korean Immigrants in the United States

In a sample of 100 older Korean immigrants residing in Los Angeles, 34 percent indicated seeing or hearing about at least one incident of elder abuse and neglect among their Korean relatives, friends, and neighbors, amounting to 46 incidents (Chang and Moon, 1997). Financial exploitation was found to be the most frequently occurring type of abuse (36 percent), followed by psychological abuse (24 percent), culturally specific types of abuse such as "grown-up children refusing to live with their parents," "lack of contact from grown-up children," etc. (17 percent), neglect (15 percent), and physical abuse (4 percent).

Cultural Considerations

A handful of research studies have looked into how different cultural groups in Asia define elder mistreatment. As is evident, Asians identify culturally specific forms of mistreatment that differ from Western perspectives. The concept of "disrespect" captures actions and attitudes that violate basic Asian cultural norms of values and behaviors. Based on a qualitative study of home care workers, Tam and Neysmith (2006) reported that "disrespect" is the key form of elder abuse in the Chinese community. Examples of disrespect in this study include "family members being excessively bossy or rude," or living in more than one place like "a ball being kicked around among relatives." Qualitative interviews with older Chinese confirmed that disrespect results in unsettling feelings in older persons; examples provided by Chinese elders included "being ignored by children" and "behaving as if (the elder person is) the enemy" (Dong et al., 2011b). In Hong Kong Chinese elders, "being treated as if transparent" is considered a serious and common form of elder abuse (Hong Kong Christian Service, 2004).

Disrespect and lack of dignified living is also considered a major form of elder abuse by older Indians (Nagpaul, 1998; Help Age India, 2012). "Being taken for granted," "being used as additional domestic help," and "not being appreciated for contributions made in household chores" are other examples of elder abuse in India (Shah et al., 1995). In many circumstances, however, abuse incidents were attributed to the lifestyles in the younger generations that do not meet the expectations of their parents (Nagpaul, 1998).

Similar observations have been made in other Asian cultures. Chang and Moon (1997) found that older Koreans consider lack of respect for and inappropriate treatments of elders by family members a prominent form of abuse. Korean elders tend to see insufficient attention from their daughters-in-law as a form of abuse. Some of the culturally specific examples of abuse include "failure to employ Korean language usage that denotes respect," "direct expression of disagreement with the mother-in-law," and "failure to acknowledge the elderly upon arriving and leaving the residence." Studies on older Japanese provided another example of culturally specific types of elder abuse. When asked to generate examples of extreme abuse, respondents provided examples of "blaming," that is, elderly parents being blamed for whatever problems the adult children were having (Arai, 2006).

Discussions

As is obvious, huge variation is observed in the reported rates of elder abuse and can be partly attributed to the methodological difference across studies.

Although most researchers have agreed on the definitions of elder abuse, many investigate different types of abuse in their studies. Some researchers include neglect and self-neglect in their studies, while many do not. To obtain more comparable results, a more consistent categorization of abuse is needed. Also contributing to the variation in prevalence estimates is the recall period used in these studies, which included 1 month, 6 months, and 1 year. With the variations in the recall period, it is extremely difficult to draw meaningful conclusions from the estimates obtained in these studies. To date, a majority of the studies on elder abuse are based on samples of non-representative groups such as clinical populations or members of community centers. They may not reflect the actual prevalence of abuse due to their small sample size and biased sample characteristics. It is observed that studies using representative samples generally reported lower rates as compared to those from non-representative samples.

This trend has several possible reasons. First, given the higher rates of abuse in older persons with physical or cognitive problems and their overrepresentation in the clinical samples, rates obtained in clinical samples are likely to be higher than those obtained from representative community samples. Second, older persons who were abused may be more inclined in participate in the research, resulting in higher rates being observed in convenience samples as compared to representative samples.

An argument has often been that much of the screening and assessment instruments developed in "Western societies" may not be able to capture culture-specific forms of elder abuse in Asian cultures. While developing local assessment tools may solve this problem, the downside of solely relying on a locally developed measure is that it would hamper efforts for cross-cultural comparison. Although it is desirable to use instruments that tap into culturally specific types of abuse, it is also essential to maintain some degree of similarity in instruments used so as to aid cross-cultural comparative studies. Furthermore, despite the fact that culturally specific types of abuse, such as disrespect or ignoring, have been identified, little is known regarding the impact of such forms of abuse. It would be desirable to compare the impacts of culturally specific forms of abuse with traditional types of abuse.

Another observation is that studies using older persons or caregivers as informants found much higher rates than those using clinicians as informants. While older persons subjected to physical violence and neglect may present with physical injuries or other observable characteristics, such as malnutrition or dehydration, those who suffered emotional abuse or financial abuse may have no presenting symptoms at all. This may also be the reason why physical violence is overrepresented in clinician-identified cases. Contrary to the common perception that perpetrators are unwilling to admit to abusive behaviors, several studies using caregivers as informants found prevalence rates comparable to those of victim reports. Further research should compare the prevalence rates of reports from different informants in order to achieve a comprehensive picture of the actual rates of abuse.

Cultural sensitivity is essential for research into elder abuse in Asia. It goes beyond using culturally sensitive instruments that measure cultural-specific types of abuse. As discussed earlier, many older Asians may be reluctant to report their own abusive experience to a person outside of their families. In conducting research, special attention should be paid in building rapport with participants in the data collection process. Studies that employed indirect estimates, for example, by asking participants to report abuse incidents that they have heard of or witnessed, may be an alternative to traditional research that directly asks participants about their abusive experience.

Research into elder abuse in Asia remains underrepresented in the literature. Part of the reason is that scholars seldom publish in international journals. In searching the literature, the author was aware that a sizable amount of work in elder abuse in Asia was published as research reports in Korean and Japanese. Scholars conducting research on elder abuse in Asia should be encouraged to publish in international English journals to disseminate their knowledge.

REFERENCES

Acierno, R., M. A. Hernandez, A. B. Amstadter, H. S. Resnick, K. Steve, W. Muzzy, and D. G. Kilpatrick. 2010. Prevalence and correlates of emotional, physical, sexual, and financial abuse and potential neglect in the United States: The National Elder Mistreatment Study. *American Journal of Public Health* 100(2):292-297.

Akaza, K., Y. Bunai, M. Tsujinaka, I. Nakamura, A. Nagai, Y. Tsukata, and I. Ohya. 2003. Elder abuse and neglect: Social problems revealed from 15 autopsy cases. *Legal Medicine* 5(1):7.

Anme, T. 2004. A study of elder abuse and risk factors in Japanese families: Focused on the social affiliation model. *Geriatrics and Gerontology International* 4:62-63.

Anme, T., M. McCall, and T. Tatara. 2005. An exploratory study of abuse among frail elders using services in a small village in Japan. *Journal of Elder Abuse & Neglect* 17(2):1-20.

Arai, M. 2006. Elder abuse in Japan. *Educational Gerontology* 32:13-23.

Bambawale, U. 1997. The abused elderly. *Indian Journal of Medical Research* 106:389-395.

Barker, J. C. 2009. Between humans and ghosts: The decrepit elderly in a Polynesian society. In *The culture context of aging: Worldwide perspectives*, edited by J. Sokolovsky. Westport, CT: Praeger.

Barnes, J. S., and C. E. Bennett. 2002. *The Asian population: 2000*. Washington, DC: U.S. Census Bureau.

Bartley, M., D. O'Neill, P. Knight, and J. O'Brien. 2011. Self-neglect and elder abuse: Related phenomena. *Journal of the American Geriatrics Society* 59(11):2163-2168.

Beach, S. R., R. Schulz, H. B. Degenholtz, N. G. Castle, J. Rosen, A. R. Foz, and R. K. Morycz. 2010. Using audio computer-assisted self-interviewing and interactive voice response to measure elder mistreatment in older adults: Feasibility and effects on prevalence estimates. *Journal of Official Statistics* 26:507-533.

Bennett, C. E., and B. Martin. 1995. *The nation's Asian and Pacific Islander population*. Washington, DC: U.S. Census Bureau.

Biolsi, T. 2001. *Deadliest enemies: Law and the making of race relations on and off Rosebud Reservation*. Berkeley: University of California Press.

Biolsi, T. 2005. Imagined geographies: Sovereignty, indigenous space, and American Indian struggle. *American Ethnologist* 32(2):239-259.

Bitondo Dyer, C., C. Toronjo, M. Cunningham, N. A. Festa, V. N. Pavlik, D. J. Hyman, E. L. Poythress, and N. S. Searle. 2005. The key elements of elder neglect: A survey of Adult Protective Service workers. *Journal of Elder Abuse & Neglect* 17(4):1-10.

Brown, A. S. 1989. A survey on elder abuse at one Native American tribe. *Journal of Elder Abuse and Neglect* 1(2):17-37.

Brown, A. S., R. C. Fernandez, and T. M. Griffith. 1990. *Service provider perceptions of elder abuse among the Navajo (Research Report RR-90-3)*. Flagstaff: Northern Arizona University Social Research Laboratory.

Buchwald, D., S. Tomita, S. Ashton, R. Furman, and S. M. Manson. 2000. Physical abuse of urban Native Americans. *Journal of General Internal Medicine* 15:562-564.

Bureau of Indian Affairs. 2013. *U.S. Department of the Interior 2013*. http://www.bia.gov/WhoWeAre/index.htm (accessed May 21, 2013).

Casado, B. L., and P. Leung. 2001. Migratory grief and depression among elderly Chinese American immigrants. *Journal of Gerontological Work* 36(1-2):5-26.

Castle, N., and S. Beach. 2013. Elder abuse in assisted living. *Journal of Applied Gerontology* 32:248-267.

CDC (Centers for Disease Control and Prevention). 2010a. *Suicide: Facts at a glance*. Atlanta, GA: CDC.

CDC. 2010b. *Web-based Injury Statistics Query and Reporting System (WISQARS)*. http://www.cdc.gov/injury/wisqars/index.html (accessed September 10, 2013).

Censky, A. 2011. *Older Americans are 47 times richer than young*. http://money.cnn.com/2011/11/07/news/economy/wealth_gap_age/index.htm (accessed September 10, 2013).

Cham, G. W., and E. Seow. 2000. The pattern of elderly abuse presenting to an emergency department. *Singapore Medical Journal* 41(12):571-574.

Chang, E., M. A. Simon, and X. Dong. 2010. Integrating cultural humility into health care professional education and training. *Advances in Health Sciences Education* [Epub ahead of print].

Chang, J., and A. Moon. 1997. Korean American elderly's knowledge and perceptions of elder abuse: A qualitative analysis of cultural factors. *Journal of Multicultural Social Work* 6:139-155.

Chao, Y. R. 1976. *Aspects of Chinese sociolinguistics: Essays by Yuen Ren Chao.* Stanford, CA: Stanford University Press.

Chokkanathan, S., and A. E. Y. Lee. 2005. Elder mistreatment in urban India: A community-based study. *Journal of Elder Abuse & Neglect* 17(2)45-61.

Chou, R. J. 2010. Filial piety by contract? The emergence, implementation, and implications of the "family support agreement" in China. *Gerontologist* 51(1):3-16.

Cisler, J. M., A. B. Amstadter, A. M. Begle, M. Hernandez, and R. Acierno. 2010. Elder mistreatment and physical health among older adults: The South Carolina Elder Mistreatment Study. *Journal of Traumatic Stress* 23(4):461-467.

Clancy, M., B. McDaid, D. O'Neill, and J. O'Brien. 2011. National profiling of elder abuse referrals. *Age and Aging* 40(3):346-352.

CMS (Centers for Medicare & Medicaid Services). 2010. *Nursing home data compendium. 2010.* Washington, DC: Centers for Medicare & Medicaid Services.

CMS. 2013. *Physician quality reporting system.* http://www.cms.gov/Medicare/Quality-Initiatives-Patient-Assessment-Instruments/PQRS/index.html?redirect=/PQRS (accessed September 10, 2013).

Collins, K. A., and S. E. Presnell. 2007. Elder neglect and the pathophysiology of aging. *American Journal of Forensic Medicine and Pathology* 28(2):157-162.

Cooper, C., A. Selwood, and G. Livingston. 2008. The prevalence of elder abuse and neglect: A systematic review. *Age and Ageing* 37(2):151-160.

Cristancho, S., D. M. Garces, K. E. Peters, and B. C. Mueller. 2008. Listening to rural Hispanic immigrants in the Midwest: A community-based participatory assessment of major barriers to health care access and use. *Qualitative Health Research* 18(5):633-646.

DeLiema, M., Z. D. Gassoumis, D. C. Homeier, and K. H. Wilber. 2012. Determining prevalence and correlates of elder abuse using promotores: Low-income immigrant Latinos report high rates of abuse and neglect. *Journal of the American Geriatrics Society* 60:1333-1339.

Dong, X. 2005. Medical implications of elder abuse and neglect. *Clinics in Geriatric Medicine* 21(2):293-313.

Dong, X. 2008. A descriptive study of sex differences in psychosocial factors and elder mistreatment in a Chinese community population. *International Journal of Gerontology* 2(4):206-214.

Dong, X. 2012. Advancing the field of elder abuse: Future directions and policy implications. *Journal of the American Geriatrics Society* 60:2151-2156.

Dong, X., and M. A. Simon. 2008. Is greater social support a protective factor against elder mistreatment? *Gerontology* 54(6):381-388.

Dong, X., and M. A. Simon. 2010. Is impairment in physical function associated with increased risk of elder mistreatment? Findings from a community-dwelling Chinese population. *Public Health Reports* 125:743-753.

Dong, X. Q., and M. A. Simon. 2013. Elder abuse as a risk factor for hospitalization in older persons. *Journal of the American Medical Association* 173(10):911-917.

Dong, X., M. A. Simon, and M. Gorbien. 2007a. Elder abuse and neglect in an urban Chinese population. *Journal of Elder Abuse & Neglect* 19(3-4):79-96.

Dong, X., M. A. Simon, M. Gorbien, J. Percak, and R. Golden. 2007b. Loneliness in older Chinese adults: A risk factor for elder mistreatment. *Journal of the American Geriatrics Society* 55(11):1831-1835.

Dong, X., M. Simon, C. Mendes de Leon, T. Fulmer, T. Beck, L. Hebert, C. Dyer, G. Paveza, and D. Evans. 2009. Elder self-neglect and abuse and mortality risk in a community-dwelling population. *Journal of the American Medical Association* 302(5):517-526.

Dong, X., M. Simon, T. Fulmer, C. F. Mendes de Leon, B. Rajan, and D. A. Evans. 2010a. Physical function decline and the risk of elder self-neglect in a community-dwelling population. *Gerontologist* 50(3):316-326.

Dong, X. Q., M. Simon, and D. Evans. 2010b. Cross-sectional study of the characteristics of reported elder self-neglect in a community-dwelling population: Findings from a population-based cohort. *Gerontology* 56(3):325-334.

Dong, X., E. Chang, E. Wong, and M. Simon. 2011a. Sustaining community–university partnerships: Lessons learned from a participatory research project with elderly Chinese. *Gateways International Journal of Community Research & Engagement* 4.

Dong, X., E. Chang, E. Wong, B. Wong, and M. A. Simon. 2011b. How do U.S. Chinese older adults view elder mistreatment? Findings from a community-based participatory research study. *Journal of Aging and Health* 23(2):289-312.

Dong, X., E. S. Chang, E. Wong, and M. Simon. 2011c. Working with culture: Lessons learned from a community-engaged project in a Chinese aging population. *Aging Health* 7(4):529-537.

Dong, X., M. A. Simon, T. Fulmer, C. F. Mendes de Leon, L. E. Hebert, and D. A. Evans. 2011d. A prospective population-based study of differences in elder self-neglect and mortality between black and white older adults. *Journals of Gerontology Series A: Biological Sciences and Medical Sciences* 66A:695-704.

Dong, X., E. Chang, E. Wong, and M. Simon. 2012a. The perceptions, social determinants, and negative health outcomes associated with depressive symptoms among U.S. Chinese older adults. *Gerontologist* 52(5):650-663.

Dong, X., E. S. Chang, E. Wong, and M. Simon. 2012b. Perception and negative effect of loneliness in a Chicago Chinese population of older adults. *Archives of Gerontology and Geriatrics* 54(1):151-159.

Dong, X., M. Simon, and D. Evans. 2012c. A population-based study of physical function and risk for elder abuse reported to social service agency: Findings from the Chicago Health and Aging Project. *Journal of Applied Gerontology* [Epub September 17].

Dong, X., Simon, M. A., and Evans, D. A. 2012d. Prospective study of the elder self-neglect and emergency department use in a community population. *American Journal of Emergency Medicine* 30:553-561.

Dyer, C. B., M. S. Gleason, K. P. Murphy, V. N. Pavlik, B. Portal, T. Regev, and D. J. Hyman. 1999. Treating elder neglect: Collaboration between a geriatrics assessment team and adult protective services. *Southern Medical Journal* 92(2):242-244.

Dyer, C. B., J. S. Goodwin, S. Pickens-Pace, J. Burnett, and P. A. Kelly. 2007. Self-neglect among the elderly: A model based on more than 500 patients seen by a geriatric medicine team. *American Journal of Public Health* 97(9):1671-1676.

Eldercare Workforce Alliance. 2013. Geriatric workforce shortage: A looming crisis for our families. Eldercare Workforce Alliance. http://www.eldercareworkforce.org/research/issuebriefs (accessed January 12, 2014).

Finance Committee, U.S. Senate. 2002. *Elder mistreatment in aging America: An urgent need for research. Panel to review risk and prevalence of elder abuse and neglect*. 107th Congress (Second Session).

Foo, L. 2003. *Asian American women: Issues, concerns, and responsive human and civil rights advocacy*. Lincoln, NE: IUniverse.

Fulmer, T., and J. Ashley. 1989. Clinical indicators of elderly neglect. *Applied Nursing Research* 2(4):161-167.

Fulmer, T., and V. M. Cahill. 1984. Assessing elder abuse: A study. *Journal of Gerontological Nursing* 10(12):16-20.

Fulmer, T., and L. C. Degutis. 1992. Elderly patients in the emergency department. *AACN Clinical Issues in Critical Care Nursing* 3(1):89-97.

Fulmer, T., D. J. McMahon, M. Baer-Hines, and B. Forget. 1992. Abuse, neglect, abandonment, violence, and exploitation: An analysis of all elderly patients seen in one emergency department during a six-month period. *Journal of Emergency Nursing* 18(6):505-510.

Fulmer, T., G. Paveza, I. Abraham, and S. Fairchild. 2000. Elder neglect assessment in the emergency department. *Journal of Emergency Nursing* 26(5):436-443.

Fulmer, T., G. Paveza, C. Vandeweerd, S. Fairchild, L. Guadagno, M. Bolton-Blatt, and R. Norman. 2005a. Dyadic vulnerability and risk profiling for elder neglect. *Gerontologist* 45(4):525-535.

Fulmer, T., G. Paveza, C. Vandeweerd, L. Guadagno, S. Fairchild, R. Norman, I. Abraham, and M. Bolton-Blatt. 2005b. Neglect assessment in urban emergency departments and confirmation by an expert clinical team. *Journal of Gerontology: Medical Sciences* 60A(8):1002-1006.

GAO (Government Accountability Office). 2011. *Elder justice: Stronger federal leadership could enhance national response to elder abuse.* http://aging.senate.gov/events/hr230kb2.pdf (accessed July 1, 2011).

GAO. 2012. Elder justice: National strategy needed to effectively combat elder financial exploitation: Report to congressional requesters. Washington, DC: Government Printing Office. http://purl.fdlp.gov/GPO/gpo33450 (accessed April 20, 2013).

Garrison, D. R. 2000. Theoretical challenges for distance education in the 21st century. *International Review of Research in Open & Distance Learning* 1(1).

Glascock, A. 2009. Is killing necessarily murder? Moral questions surrounding assisted suicide and death. In *The cultural context of aging: Worldwide perspectives*, 3rd ed., edited by J. Sokolovsky. Westport, CT: Praeger Publishers.

Godkin, M. A., R. S. Wolf, and K. A. Pillemer. 1989. A case-comparison analysis of elder abuse and neglect. *International Journal of Aging and Human Development* 28(3):207-225.

Gunther, J. 2011. *The Utah cost of financial exploitation.* http://www.dhs.utah.gov/pdf/utah-financial-exploitation-study.pdf (accessed April 20, 2013).

Guo, Z. 2000. *Ginseng and aspirin: Health care alternatives for aging Chinese in New York.* Ithaca, NY: Cornell University Press.

Harrell, R., C. H. Toronjo, J. McLaughlin, V. N. Pavlik, D. J. Hyman, and C. B. Dyer. 2002. How geriatricians identify elder abuse and neglect. *American Journal of the Medical Sciences* 323(1):34-38.

HelpAge India. 2012. *Elder abuse in India: Summary of research reports.* http://www.helpageindia.org/pdf/Report_Elder-Abuse_India2012.pdf (accessed September 10, 2013).

HelpAge International. 2013. *Global agewatch 2013 insights report.* London, UK: HelpAge International.

Holkup, P. A., E. M. Salois, T. Tripp-Reimer, and C. Weinert. 2007. Drawing on wisdom from the past: An elder abuse intervention with tribal communities. *Gerontologist* 47(2):248-254.

Hong Kong Christian Service. 2004. *Elder abuse in Hong Kong.* http://www.hkcs.org/archives/ears/ears-e.html (accessed September 10, 2013).

Hudson, M. F., and J. R. Carlson. 1999. Elder abuse: Its meaning to Caucasians, African Americans, and Native Americans. In *Understanding elder abuse in minority populations*, edited by T. Tatara. Philadelphia, PA: Brunner/Mazel. Pp. 187-204.

Ikels, C. 2004. *Filial piety: Practice and discourse in contemporary East Asia.* Stanford, CA: Stanford University Press.

Israel, B. A. 2000. Community-based participatory research: Principles, rationale and policy recommendations. In *Successful models of community-based participatory research*. Washington, DC: National Institutes of Health. Pp. 16-22.

Jackson, S. L., and T. L.Hafemeister. 2013. Understanding elder abuse: New directions for developing theories. *National Institute of Justice Research in Brief*. Washington, DC: U.S. Department of Justice.

Jervis, L. L., and AI-SUPERPFP Team. 2009. Disillusionment, faith, and cultural traumatization on a Northern Plains reservation. *Traumatology* 15(1):11-22.

Jervis, L. L., P. Spicer, S. M. Manson, and AI-SUPERPFP Team. 2003. Boredom, "trouble," and postcolonial reservation life. *Ethos* 31(1):38-58.

Jervis, L. L., M. Boland, and A. Fickenscher. 2010. American Indian family caregivers' experiences with helping elders. *Journal of Cross-Cultural Gerontology* 25(4):355-369.

Jervis, L. L., A. Fickenscher, J. Beals, and the Shielding American Indian Elders Project Team. 2013. Assessment of elder mistreatment in two American Indian samples: Psychometric characteristics of the HS-EAST and the native elder life financial exploitation and neglect measures. *Journal of Applied Gerontology* 32(7).

Jervis, L. L., W. Sconzert-Hall, and Shielding American Indian Elders Team. In preparation. *Conceptualizations of mistreatment among American Indian elders*.

Kaasaslainen, S., D. Craig, and D. Wells. 2000. Impact of the Caring for Aging Relatives Group Program: An evaluation. *Public Health Nursing* 17(3):169-177.

Karlawish, J. 2013. *Elder abuse and neglect: Ethical consideration in research and care*. Presented at Elder Abuse and Its Prevention: A Workshop. Washington, DC: Institute of Medicine, April 17.

Keskinoglu, P., M. Pýcakcýefe, N. Bilgic, H. Giray, N. Karakus, and R. Ucku. 2007. Elder abuse and neglect in two different socioeconomic districts in Izmir, Turkey. *International Psychogeriatrics* 19(4):719-731.

Kim, O., H. O. Jeon, and B. H. Im. 2012. The relating factors of elder abuse among community-dwelling elderly with stroke. *Korean Journal of Adult Nursing* 24:466-476.

Kishimoto, Y., S. Terada, N. Takeda, E. Oshima, H. Honda, H. Yoshida, O. Yokota, and Y. Uchitomi. 2013. Abuse of people with cognitive impairment by family caregivers in Japan (a cross-sectional study). *Psychiatry Research* S0165-S1781(13):46-52.

Kleinman, A., L. Eisenberg, and B. Good. 1978. Culture, illness and care: Clinical lessons from anthropologic and cross-cultural research. *Annals of Internal Medicine* 88:251-256.

Lachs, M. S., C. Williams, S. O'Brien, L. Hurst, and R. Horwitz. 1996. Older adults. An 11-year longitudinal study of Adult Protective Service use. *Archives of Internal Medicine* 156(4):449-453.

Lachs, M. S., C. Williams, S. O'Brien, L. Hurst, and R. I. Horwitz. 1997. Risk factors for reported elder abuse and neglect: A nine-year observational cohort study. *Gerontologist* 37(4):469-474.

Lachs, M. S., C. S. Williams, S. O'Brien, and K. A. Pillemer. 2002. Adult Protective Service use and nursing home placement. *Gerontologist* 42(6):734-739.

Lachs, M., R. Bachman, C. S. Williams, and J. R. O'Leary. 2007. Resident-to-resident elder mistreatment and police contact in nursing homes: Findings from a population-based cohort. *Journal of the American Geriatrics Society* 55(6):840-845.

Lai, D. W. 2011. Abuse and neglect experienced by aging Chinese in Canada. *Journal of Elder Abuse & Neglect* 23(4):326-347.

Lan, P. 2002. Subcontracting filial piety—elder care in ethnic Chinese immigrant families in California. *Journal of Family Issues* 23(7):812-835.

Laumann, E. O., S. A. Leitsch, and L. J. Waite. 2008. Elder mistreatment in the United States: Prevalence estimates from a nationally representative study. *Journal of Gerontology: Social Sciences* 63B:S248-S254.

Lee, M., and S. R. Kolomer. 2005. Caregiver burden, dementia, and elder abuse in South Korea. *Journal of Elder Abuse & Neglect* 17(1):61-74.

Leng, S. X., X. P. Tian, and S. Durso. 2008. The aging population and development of geriatrics in China. *Journal of the American Geriatrics Society* 56(3):379-381.

Lifespan of Greater Rochester, Inc., Weill Cornell Medical Center of Cornell University, and New York City Department for the Aging. 2011. Under the radar: New York State Elder Abuse Prevalence Study. In *Self-reported prevalence and documented case surveys*. New York: New York State Office of Children and Family Services.

Liu, W. T., and E. Yu. 1985. Asian/Pacific American elderly: Mortality differentials, health status, and use of health services. *Journal of Applied Gerontology* 4(1):35-64.

Lok, D. 2012. New protocol brings access to justice to older adults in New York City. *New York Law Journal* 1(8).

Martinez, I. L., O. Carter-Pokras, and P. B. Broan. 2009. Addressing the challenges of Latino health research: Participatory approaches in an emergent urban community. *Journal of the National Medical Association* 101(9):908-914.

Maxwell, E. K., and R. J. Maxwell. 1992. Insults to the body civil: Mistreatment of elderly in two Plains Indian tribes. *Journal of Cross-Cultural Gerontology* 7:3-23.

McCrae, R. R., and P. T. J. Costa. 1987. Validation of the five-factor model of personality across instruments and observers. *Journal of Personality and Social Psychology* 52(1):81-90.

McDonald, L., and C. Thomas. 2013. Elder abuse through a life course lens. *International Psychogeriatrics* (8):1235-1243.

McDonald, P. L. 2011. Elder abuse and neglect in Canada: The glass is still half full. *Canadian Journal on Aging/La Revue Canadienne du Vieillissement* 30(3):1-30.

McKee, L. 2010. Digital maps: An essential part of every citizen's interface to the n11. *An Open GIS Consortium White Paper*. http://www.portal.opengeospatial.org/files/?artifact_id=6199 (accessed January 12, 2014).

McMullen, T., and K. Schwartz. 2013. *The CMS elder maltreatment and care symposium*. Baltimore, MD: Centers for Medicaid & Medicare Services. March 8.

Mencius, D. C. Lau. 2005. *Mencius*. London, England: Penguin Classics.

MetLife Mature Market Institute. 2011. The MetLife study of elder financial abuse. https://www.metlife.com/assets/cao/mmi/publications/studies/2011/Highlights/mmi-elder-financial-abuse-highlights.pdf (accessed September 10, 2013).

Minkler, M. 2005. Community-based research partnerships: Challenges and opportunities. *Journal of Urban Health* 82(2):ii3-ii12.

Minkler, M., and N. Wallerstein. 2003. *Community-based participatory research for health*. San Francisco, CA: Jossey-Bass.

Moon, A., and O. Williams. 1993. Perceptions of elder abuse and help-seeking patterns among African-American, Caucasian American, and Korean-American elderly women. *Gerontologist* 33(3):386-395.

Moon, A., S. Tomita, and S. Jung-Kamei. 2002. Elder mistreatment among four Asian American groups: An exploratory study on tolerance, victim blaming and attitudes toward third party intervention. *Journal of Gerontological Social Work* 36(1-2):153-169.

Moreno-John, G., A. Gachie, C. M. Fleming, A. Napoles-Springer, E. Mutran, and S. M. Manson. 2004. Ethnic minority older adults participating in clinical research: Developing trust. *Journal of Aging and Health* 16:93-123.

Mosqueda, L., and X. Dong. 2011. Elder abuse and self-neglect: "I don't care anything about going to the doctors . . . to be honest." *Journal of the American Medical Association* (306):532-540.

Mosqueda, L., K. Burnight, and S. Liao. 2005. The life cycle of bruises in older adults. *American Geriatrics Society* 53:1339-1343.

Mui, A. C. 1996. Depression among elderly Chinese immigrants: An exploratory study. *Social Work* 41(6):633-645.
Nagpaul, K. 1998. Elder abuse among Asian Indians: Traditional versus modern perspectives. *Journal of Elder Abuse & Neglect* 9:77-92.
Nakanishi, M., Y. Hoshishiba, N. Iwama, T. Okada, E. Kato, and H. Takahashi. 2009. Impact of the elder abuse prevention and caregiver support law on system development among municipal governments in Japan. *Health Policy* 90(2-3):254-261.
Nakanishi, M., T. Nakashima, and T. Honda. 2010. Disparities in systems development for elder abuse prevention among municipalities in Japan: Implications for strategies to help municipalities develop community systems. *Social Science & Medicine* 71(2):400-404.
National Center on Elder Abuse. 1998. *The National Elder Abuse Incidence Study: Final Report.* Prepared for the Administration on Aging in collaboration with Westat, Inc.
National Center on Elder Abuse. 1999. *Attitudes toward elder mistreatment and reporting: A multicultural study.* Washington, DC: National Center on Elder Abuse.
National Center on Elder Abuse. 2013. *Types of abuse.* http://www.ncea.aoa.gov/FAQ/Type_ Abuse (accessed April 20, 2013).
National Committee for the Prevention of Elder Abuse. 2008. *Financial abuse.* http://www.preventelderabuse.org/elderabuse/fin_abuse.html (accessed September 10, 2013).
National Indian Council on Aging. 2004. *A review of the literature—elder abuse in Indian country: Research, policy, and practice* Washington, DC: National Center on Elder Abuse.
Neale, A. V., M. A. Hwalek, R. O. Scott, M. C Sengstock, and C. Stahl. 1991. Validation of the Hwalek-Sengstock Elder Abuse Screening Test. *Journal of Applied Gerontology* 10:406-418.
Ng, A. C. Y., D. R. Phillips, and W. K.-m. Lee. 2002. Persistence and challenges to filial piety and informal support of older persons in a modern Chinese society: A case study in Tuen Mun, Hong Kong. *Journal of Aging Studies* 16(2):135-153.
NIEJI (National Indigenous Elder Justice Initiative). 2013. *National Indigenous Elder Justice Initiative (NIEJI).* http://www.nieji.org (accessed May 23, 2013).
Norman, J. 1988. *Chinese.* Cambridge, England: Cambridge University Press.
NRC (National Research Council). 2003. *Elder mistreatment: Abuse, neglect, and exploitation in an aging America.* Washington, DC: The National Academies Press.
O'Brien, J., C. Collins, A. Niriain, V. Long, and D. O'Neill. 2013a. Elder abuse and neglect: A survey of Irish general practitioners. *Journal of Elder Abuse and Neglect* [Epub August 5, 2013].
O'Brien, J., C. Cooney, M. Bartley, and D. O'Neill. 2013b. Self-neglect: A survey of old age psychiatrists in Ireland. *International Psychogeriatrics* [Epub July 5, 2013].
Office of the Assistant Secretary for Planning and Evaluation. 2010. Congressional report on the feasibility of establishing a uniform national database on elder abuse. Washington, DC: Department of Health and Human Services.
Oh, J., H. S. Kim, et al. 2006. A study of elder abuse in Korea. *International Journal of Nursing Studies* 43:203-214.
Parikh, N. S., M. C. Fahs, D. Shelley, and R. Yerneni. 2009. Health behaviors of older Chinese adults living in New York City. *Journal of Community Health* 34:6-15.
Pavlik, V. N., D. J. Hyman, N. A. Festa, and C. Bitondo Dyer. 2001. Quantifying the problem of abuse and neglect in adults—analysis of a statewide database. *Journal of the American Geriatrics Society* 49(1):45-48.
Perez-Rojo, G., M. Izal, M. T. Sancho, and Grupo de Investigación Trátame Bien. 2010. Linguistic and cultural adaptation of two tools for detecting suspected elder abuse. *Revista Española de Geriatría y Gerontología* 45(4):213-218.

Phua, D. H., T. W. Ng, and E. Seow. 2008. Epidemiology of suspected elderly mistreatment in Singapore. *Singapore Medical Journal* 49(10):765-773.

Pillemer, K. A., and D. Finkelhor. 1988. The prevalence of elder abuse: A random sample survey. *Gerontologist* 28(1):51-57.

Podnieks, E. 1999. Support groups for abused older adults. In *Elder abuse work: Best practice in Britain and Canada*, edited by J. Pritchard. London, England: Jessica Kingsley Publications.

Podnieks, E. 2002. Abuse of the elderly. In *World report on violence and health*, edited by E. Krug, et al. Geneva, Switzerland: World Health Organization.

Podnieks, E., G. J. Anetzberger, and P. B. Teaster. 2010. Worldview environmental scan on elder abuse. *Journal of Elder Abuse & Neglect* 22:161-179.

Quality Insights Pennsylvania. 2013. PQRS specification #181: Elder maltreatment screening and follow-up plan. Washington, DC: CMS.

Red Horse, J. 1983. Indian family values and experiences. In *The psychosocial development of minority group children*, edited by G. J. Powell. New York: Brunner/Mazel. Pp. 258-271.

Red Horse, J. 1997. Traditional American Indian family systems. *Families, Systems, & Health* 15(3):243-250.

Rittman, M., L. B. Kuzmeskus, and M. A. Flum. 1999. A synthesis of current knowledge on minority elder abuse. In *Understanding elder abuse in minority populations*, edited by T. Tatara. Philadelphia, PA: Brunner/Mazel. Pp. 221-238.

Russell, S. L., T. Fulmer, G. Singh, M. Valenti, R. Vermula, and S. M. Strauss. 2012. Screening for elder mistreatment in a dental clinic population. *Journal of Elder Abuse & Neglect* 24(4):326-339.

Sasaki, M., Y. Arai, K. Kumamoto, K. Abe, A. Arai, and Y. Mizuno. 2007. Factors related to potentially harmful behaviors towards disabled older people by family caregivers in Japan. *International Journal of Geriatric Psychiatry* 22(3):250-257.

Schweitzer, M. M. 1999. *American Indian grandmothers: Traditions and transitions*. Albuquerque: University of New Mexico Press.

Sebastian, D., and T. V. Sekher. 2011. Extent and nature of elder abuse in Indian families: A study in Kerala. *HelpAge India Research and Development Journal* 17:20-28.

Shah, G., R. Veedon, and S. Vasi. 1995. Elder abuse in India. *Journal of Elder Abuse & Neglect* 6:101-118.

Shields, L. B. E., D. M. Hunsaker, and J. C. Hunsaker. 2004. Abuse and neglect: A ten-year review of mortality and morbidity in our elders in a large metropolitan area. *Journal of Forensic Sciences* 49(1):122-127.

Shinagawa, L. 2008. *A portrait of Chinese Americans*. Asian American Studies Program, University of Maryland, College Park.

Sue, S., N. Zane, G. C. N. Hall, and L. K. Berger. 2009. The case for cultural competency in psychotherapeutic interventions. *Annual Review of Psychology* 60:525-548.

Tam, S., and S. Neysmith. 2006. Disrespect and isolation: Elder abuse in Chinese communities. *Canadian Journal on Aging* 25(2):141-151.

Tervalon, M. 2003. Components of culture in health for medical students' education. *Academic Medicine* 78(6):570-576.

Tsai, J. H. 1999. Meaning of filial piety in the Chinese parent–child relationship: Implications for culturally competent health care. *Journal of Cultural Diversity* 6(1):26-34.

Tsukada, N., Y. Saito, and T. Tatara. 2001. Japanese older people's perceptions of "elder abuse." *Journal of Elder Abuse & Neglect* 13(1):71-89.

U.S. Census Bureau. 2009. *U.S. population clock projection.* http://www.census.gov/population/www.popclockus.html (accessed November 6, 2009).

U.S. Census Bureau. 2011. *2010 Census demographic profile*. Washington, DC.

U.S. Census Bureau. 2012. Facts for features: Older Americans month: May 2012. http://www.census.gov/newsroom/releases/archives/facts_for_features_special_editions/cb12-ff07.html (accessed March 1, 2012).
Wakeling, S., M. Jorgensen, S. Michaelson, and M. Begay. 2001. *Policing on American Indian reservations: A report to the National Institute of Justice.* Washington, DC: U.S. Department of Justice.
Wang, J. J. 2005. Psychological abuse behavior exhibited by caregivers in the care of the elderly and correlated factors in long-term care facilities in Taiwan. *Journal of Nursing Research* 13(4):271-280.
Wang, J. J., J. N. Lin, and F. P. Lee. 2006. Psychologically abusive behavior by those caring for the elderly in a domestic context. *Geriatric Nursing* 27:284-291.
Washington Post. 2012. A closer look at seniors' wealth. http://articles.washingtonpost.com/2012-08-16/opinions/35490880_1_senior-population-share-of-medicare-costs-medicare-tab (accessed April 20, 2013).
WHO (World Health Organization). 2002. *Missing voices: Views of older persons on elder abuse.* Geneva, Switzerland: WHO.
WHO. 2008. *A global response to elder abuse and neglect: Building primary health care capacity to deal with the problem worldwide: Main report.* Geneva, Switzerland: WHO.
Wiglesworth, A. 2010. Screening for abuse and neglect of people with dementia. *Journal of the American Geriatrics Society* 58(3):493-500.
Wiglesworth, A., L. Mosqueda, K. Burnight, T. Younglove, and D. Jeske. 2006. Findings from an elder abuse forensic center. *Gerontologist* 46(2):277-283.
Wiglesworth, A., R. Austin, M. Corona, D. Schneider, S. Liao, L. Gibbs, and L. Mosqueda. 2009. Bruising as a marker of physical elder abuse. *Journal of the American Geriatrics Society* 58:493-500.
Wiglesworth, A., L. Mosqueda, L. Mulnard, S. Liao, L. Gibbs, and W. Fitzgerald. 2010. Screening for elder abuse and neglect of people with dementia. *Journal of the American Geriatrics Society* 58:493-500.
Wood, E. F. 2006. State level adult guardianship data: An exploratory survey. *American Bar Association Commission on Law and Aging for the National Center on Elder Abuse* 11.
Wu, L., H. Chen, Y. Hu, H. Xiang, X. Yu, T. Zhang, T. and Z. Coa 2012. Prevalence and associated factors of elder mistreatment in a rural community in People's Republic of China: A cross sectional study. *PLoS ONE* 7:1-8.
Xu, Y., and B. Wang. 2007. *Ethnic minorities of China—journey into China.* China: Intercontinental Press.
Yaffe, M. J., C. Wolfson, D. Weiss, and M. Lithwick. 2008. Development and validation of a tool to assist physicians' identification of elder abuse: The Elder Abuse Suspicion Index (EASI©). *Journal of Elder Abuse & Neglect* 20(3):276-230.
Yaffe, M. J., C. Wolfson, and M. Lithwick. 2009. Professionals show different enquiry strategies for elder abuse detection: Implications for training and interprofessional care. *Journal of Interprofessional Care* 23(6):646-654.
Yaffe, M. J., M. Lithwick, and D. Weiss. 2012. Seniors' self-administration of the Elder Abuse Suspicion Index (EASI): A feasibility study. *Journal of Elder Abuse & Neglect* 24(2):277-292.
Yamada, Y. 1999. A telephone counseling program for elder abuse in Japan. *Journal of Elder Abuse & Neglect* 11:105-112.
Yan, E., and T. Kwok. 2010. Abuse of older Chinese with dementia by their family caregivers: An inquiry into the role of caregiver burden. *International Journal of Geriatric Psychiatry* 6:527-535.
Yan, E., and C. S. Tang. 2001. Prevalence and psychological impact of Chinese elder abuse. *Journal of Interpersonal Violence* 16(11):1158-1174.

Yan, E., and C. S. Tang. 2003. Proclivity to elder abuse: A community study on Hong Kong Chinese. *Journal of Interpersonal Violence* 18(9):999-1017.

Yan, E., and C. S. Tang. 2004. Elder abuse by caregivers: A study of prevalence and risk factors in Hong Kong Chinese families. *Journal of Family Violence* 19(5):269-277.

Yu, E., C. Chang, W. Liu, and S. Kan. 1985. Asian–white mortality differentials: Are there excess deaths? In *Report of the Secretary's Task Force on Black Minority Health*, edited by M. M. Heckler. Washington, DC: Department of Health and Human Services. Pp. 209-254.

Zhang, Z., C. Page, T. Conner, and L. A. Post. 2012. Family members' reports on non-staff abuse in Michigan nursing homes. *Journal of Elder Abuse and Neglect* 24:357-362.

Appendixes

Appendix A

Workshop Agenda

ELDER ABUSE AND ITS PREVENTION: A WORKSHOP
APRIL 17-18, 2013
AGENDA

> Violence and related forms of abuse against elders is a global public health and human rights problem with far-reaching consequences, resulting in increased death, disability, and exploitation with collateral effects on well-being. Data suggest that at least 10 percent of elders in the United States are victims of elder abuse every year. In low- and middle-income countries, where the burden of violence is the greatest, the figure is likely even higher. In addition, elders experiencing risk factors such as diminishing cognitive function, caregiver dependence, and social isolation are more vulnerable to maltreatment and underreporting. As the world population of adults ages 65 and older continues to grow, the implications of elder abuse for health care, social welfare, justice, and financial systems are great. However, despite the magnitude of global elder maltreatment, it has been an underappreciated public health problem.
>
> This workshop will illuminate the burden of elder abuse around the world and the evidence base for its detection and prevention. Occurrences and co-occurrences of different types of abuse—including physical, sexual, and emotional violence; neglect; and financial exploitation—will be addressed. Promising innovative approaches to intervention and prevention will be explored, as well as opportunities for scalability and cross-sectoral collaboration.

DAY 1: WEDNESDAY, APRIL 17, 2013

8:00 AM   Continental breakfast will be served

8:15 AM   Welcome
            JACQUELYN CAMPBELL, *Johns Hopkins School of Nursing, Planning Committee Co-Chair*
            XINQI DONG, *Rush Institute for Healthy Aging, Planning Committee Co-Chair*

8:30 AM   Opening Remarks
            JUDITH SALERNO, *Institute of Medicine*

8:45 AM   Keynote
            KATHY GREENLEE, *Administration for Community Living/Administration on Aging*
            CAROLE JOHNSON, *White House Domestic Policy Council*

9:15 AM   Panel I: Overview of Elder Abuse Globally

> This panel will address the global perspectives of elder abuse and the growing international recognition of its impacts on individuals, families, communities, and societies. Panelists will illuminate different types of maltreatment and their common co-occurrences, including abuse, neglect, and financial exploitation.

            Moderator: ALEXANDRE KALACHE, *International Longevity Centre–Brazil, Planning Committee*
            • GILL LIVINGSTON, *University College of London*
            • RONALD ACIERNO, *Medical University of South Carolina*
            • ELSIE YAN, *University of Hong Kong*

10:00 AM   Q&A

10:30 AM   BREAK

10:45 AM   Conceptual Framework

> This session will aim to describe the diverse conceptual frameworks proposed to examine the issues of elder abuse. Based on the literature and work of the National Academy of Sciences (NAS), Pamela Teaster will summarize key conceptual frameworks with relevance to elder abuse: ecological framework, cycle of violence framework, NAS sociocultural context framework, and lifecourse framework.

PAMELA TEASTER, *University of Kentucky*

11:05 AM   Q&A

11:15 AM   Panel II: Risk and Protective Factors and Adverse Health Outcomes

> The objectives of this session are to describe the status of evidence regarding (1) factors influencing the likelihood of elder abuse (risk factors, protective factors, correlates/comorbid conditions, etc., for victimization and perpetration, according to elder abuse type, setting, and ecological level); (2) adverse outcomes stemming from experiences that are abusive, neglectful, or exploitative; and (3) scope and factors associated with elder abuse in assisted living and long-term care settings.

Moderator: JEFFREY HALL, *Centers for Disease Control and Prevention, Planning Committee*
- ROBERT WALLACE, *University of Iowa College of Public Health*
- XINQI DONG, *Rush Institute for Healthy Aging, Planning Committee Co-Chair*
- MARK LACHS, *Weill Cornell Medical College*

12:00 PM   Q&A

12:15 PM   LUNCH

1:15 PM   Keynote
            MARIE BERNARD, *National Institute on Aging*

1:45 PM   Panel III: Neglect and Self-Neglect

> The goals of the session are to (1) review what we know about caregiver neglect and self-neglect as a subset of elder abuse; (2) examine how caregiver neglect is distinctly different from self-neglect; (3) explore what research is crucial for future progress; and (4) determine possible ways to prepare the workforce to detect, treat, and prevent caregiver neglect and self-neglect.

Moderator and Discussant: JAMES O'BRIEN, *University of Louisville*
- TERRY FULMER, *Northeastern University, Planning Committee*
- CARMEL DYER, *The University of Texas Health Sciences Center at Houston*
- KATHLEEN QUINN, *National Adult Protective Services Association*

2:30 PM   Q&A

2:45 PM   BREAK

3:00 PM   Panel IV: Ethical Considerations in Research and Practice

> What are the challenges and ethical issues in measuring and conducting research on elder abuse and implementing interventions? Panelists will discuss issues of informed consent and human subject protection, certificate of confidentiality, decisional capacity issues, lack of reporting, stigma and discrimination, and how to approach victims who refuse needed services. Consideration will be given to challenges within the United States and globally.

Moderator: BRIGID MCCAW, *Kaiser Permanente*
- SIDNEY STAHL, *National Institute on Aging (retired)*
- SUSAN LYNCH, *Department of Justice*
- JASON KARLAWISH, *University of Pennsylvania*

4:00 PM   Q&A

4:15 PM   Wrap-Up and Discussion of Day 1
           Moderator: XINQI DONG, *Rush Institute for Healthy Aging, Planning Committee Co-Chair*
           • AGNES TIWARI, *University of Hong Kong*
           • GILL LIVINGSTON, *University College of London*
           • ELIZABETH PODNIEKS, *Ryerson University*

5:15 PM   ADJOURN DAY 1

DAY 2: THURSDAY, APRIL 18, 2013

8:00 AM   Continental breakfast will be served

8:15 AM   Welcome and Recap of Day 1

8:30 AM   Keynote
           GREG SHAW, *International Federation on Ageing*

8:50 AM   Panel V: Cultural Diversity and Role of Community

> The goals of this session are to (1) understand the scope of elder abuse in diverse communities; (2) explore in depth the sociocultural context (measurement, detection, treatment, and help seeking) for elder abuse in diverse communities; (3) examine the role of grassroots community organization in prevention of elder abuse; and (4) explore the role of Community Based Participatory Research (CBPR) methodology in advancing the field of elder abuse and its prevention.

           Moderator: XINQI DONG, *Rush Institute for Healthy Aging, Planning Committee Co-Chair*
           • CHARLES MOUTON, *Meharry Medical College*
           • LORI JERVIS, *University of Oklahoma*
           • E-SHIEN CHANG, *Rush Institute for Healthy Aging*
           • JAVIER VASQUEZ, *Pan American Health Organization*

9:50 AM   Q&A

10:10 AM   BREAK

10:25 AM   Panel VI: Screening and Detection

> This panel will discuss the measurement development, screening, and prevention of elder abuse across varied settings and providers. This panel will open up with a discussion about elder maltreatment measurement work with the Centers for Medicare & Medicaid Services. Other panel discussions will explore what screening and prevention are and how to improve these processes, led by researchers in the field of elder abuse.

TARA MCMULLEN, *Centers for Medicare & Medicaid Services, Planning Committee*
KIMBERLY SCHWARTZ, *Centers for Medicare & Medicaid Services*
Respondents:
- MARK YAFFE, *McGill University*
- SCOTT BEACH, *University of Pittsburgh*

11:05 AM   Q&A

11:20 AM   Panel VII: Interventions

> Panelists will present intervention models and strategies that target different forms of elder abuse and their evidence of effectiveness and success. A moderated panel discussion will focus on opportunities for cross-sector collaboration, and adaptation and scalability of promising approaches.

Moderator: JACQUELYN CAMPBELL, *Johns Hopkins School of Nursing, Planning Committee Co-Chair*
- DANIEL REINGOLD, *The Hebrew Home at Riverdale*
- RONALD LONG, *Wells Fargo Advisors*
- LORI STIEGEL, *American Bar Association*

12:15 PM   Q&A

12:30 PM   LUNCH (Pick up lunch and head to breakout groups)

12:45 PM   BREAKOUT SESSIONS

> The purpose of the breakout sessions is to explore primary, secondary, and tertiary prevention strategies in different settings, as well as challenges and barriers to implementing such strategies. Specific focus will be given to opportunities for cross-sector collaboration and issues of potential scalability and transferability.

- Health Care System Breakout Leaders:
  MARK YAFFE, *McGill University*
  ELSIE YAN, *University of Hong Kong*

- Legal System Breakout Leaders:
  CHARLES SABATINO, *American Bar Association*
  ALEXANDRE KALACHE, *International Longevity Centre–Brazil, Planning Committee*

- Community-Based Breakout Leaders:
  JOY SOLOMON, *The Hebrew Home at Riverdale*
  JEFFREY HALL, *Centers for Disease Control and Prevention, Planning Committee*

- Financial Sector Breakout Leaders:
  PAUL SMOCER, *Financial Services Round Table/BITS*
  EDWIN WALKER, *Administration on Aging, Planning Committee*

2:00 PM   BREAK

2:15 PM   Reports from the Breakout Groups
           Moderator: KATRINA BAUM, *National Institute of Justice*

2:45 PM   Panel VIII: Health Policy and Promoting Awareness

> Often compared to the campaigns against domestic violence and child abuse, relative to incidence data and estimates, efforts to combat elder abuse are far behind the curve when it comes to development and implementation of efficient and effective responses. In the United States, passage of the Elder Justice Act as part of the Patient Protection and Affordable Care Act was a first step in solidifying federal activities dedicated to the eradication of elder abuse. This panel will address opportunities, both in the United States and globally, for policy makers and a wide range of stakeholders to identify the variety of ways that elder abuse cuts across sectors and how to promote awareness and prevention.

Moderator: EDWIN WALKER, *Administration on Aging, Planning Committee*
- SUSAN SOMERS, *International Network for the Prevention of Elder Abuse*
- MARIE-THERESE CONNOLLY, *Woodrow Wilson International Center for Scholars*
- ROBERT BLANCATO, *Elder Justice Coalition*

3:30 PM   Q&A

3:45 PM   Way Forward
KATHY GREENLEE, *Administration for Community Living/Administration on Aging*
TERRY FULMER, *Northeastern University, Planning Committee*
GREG SHAW, *International Federation on Ageing*

4:30 PM   ADJOURN DAY 2

Appendix B

Speaker Biographical Sketches

Ronald Acierno, Ph.D., is director of the Posttraumatic Stress Disorder (PTSD) Clinical Team at the Ralph H. Johnson Veterans Affairs (VA) Medical Center and professor in the Department of Psychiatry at the Medical University of South Carolina, where he is director of the Older Adult Crime Victims Clinic. In addition, he is the executive director and founder of the non-profit *Veterans on Deck*, an organization that uses sailing as a means of community reintegration for Veterans. Dr. Acierno has two related but distinct research foci: epidemiological studies of elder mistreatment and treatment outcome studies with anxiety disorders, focusing on PTSD in military, disaster-affected, and violence-affected populations. His recent research is on using home-based telemedicine for treatment delivery for victims of trauma, disaster, combat or loss, and epidemiology. Thus, Dr. Acierno mixes epidemiological research with treatment outcome research, and keeps close to the clinical world as a clinician-administrator for treatment programs serving both civilian and military traumatized populations.

Scott Beach, Ph.D., is associate director and director of the Survey Research Program at the University Center for Social and Urban Research at the University of Pittsburgh. In addition to his interests in survey methodology, research design, and statistics, Dr. Beach has interests and has published in areas such as aging and caregiver stress, elder abuse, and technology and aging. He has directed and been involved with projects funded by the National Institutes of Health (NIH) and the National Science Foundation, among many others.

Marie Bernard, M.D., is deputy director of the National Institute on Aging (NIA). Working closely with the NIA director, she oversees more than $1 billion in aging research conducted and supported annually by the Institute. As senior geriatrician, she is particularly interested in the translation of NIA research from the basic laboratory to the bedside and community, and in the pipeline of future scientists. She co-chairs the Older Adults Workgroup and the Alzheimer's and Other Dementias Workgroup for Healthy People 2020. She serves on the NIH Task Force on Women in the Biomedical Workforce, co-chairing the Women of Color Subcommittee. She also serves on the Diversity Task Force and the Bioethics Task Force. She serves as NIA's liaison to the American Federation for Aging Research, American Geriatrics Society, Department of Veteran Affairs, and Gerontological Society of America. Until 2008, Dr. Bernard was the endowed professor and founding chair of the Donald W. Reynolds Department of Geriatric Medicine at the University of Oklahoma College of Medicine. She concomitantly served as associate chief of staff for geriatrics and extended care at the Oklahoma City VA Medical Center. She has been president of the Association of Directors of Geriatric Academic Programs, president of the Association for Gerontology in Higher Education, chair of the VA National Research Advisory Committee, and chair of the Clinical Medicine (now Health Sciences) Section of the Gerontological Society of America. Her research interests include nutrition and function in aging populations, with particular emphasis on ethnic minorities. She received her undergraduate training at Bryn Mawr College, where she graduated cum laude with honors in chemistry. She earned her M.D. from the University of Pennsylvania. She trained in internal medicine at Temple University Hospital in Philadelphia, where she served as chief resident. She received additional training through the Association of American Medical Colleges (AAMC) Health Services Research Institute, the Geriatric Education Center of Pennsylvania, and the Wharton School Executive Development Program.

Robert Blancato, M.P.A., is president of Matz, Blancato and Associates, a firm founded in 1996, with offices in Washington and New York. It provides a wide array of services for clients ranging from consulting and lobbying to advocacy services and association and coalition management. Preceding this, Mr. Blancato had a career in public service spanning more than 20 years in both Congress and the Executive Branch. He was appointed by President Clinton to be executive director of the 1995 White House Conference on Aging. Ten years later, he was named to the Policy Committee for the 2005 Conference by Rep. Nancy Pelosi (D-CA). Mr. Blancato currently serves as National Coordinator of the 3,000-member nonpartisan Elder Justice Coalition. He also serves as executive director of the National Association of Nutrition and Aging Services Programs. He is the state president of AARP Virginia. As a volunteer, Mr. Blancato serves on the Board and Executive Committee of the American Society on Aging. He is also on the Board of the National Council on Aging and Generations United. He was appointed in 2008 by Governor Tim Kaine of Virginia to be on the Commonwealth Council on Aging, served as chair from 2009 to 2011, and was reappointed for another 4-year term by Governor Robert McDonnell in 2012. He has been on the adjunct faculty for a number of schools, including the New School for Social Research, George Washington University, University of Maryland, and the Brookdale Center at Hunter College. He has received a number of awards for advocacy and service, including the Arthur Flemming Award and the highest advocacy awards from the Older Women's League and the National Association of Area Agencies on Aging. In 2012 he was awarded the Riland Medal of Public Service from the New York Institute of Technology. Mr. Blancato holds a B.A. from Georgetown University and an M.P.A. from American University.

Jacquelyn C. Campbell, Ph.D., R.N. (*Forum Member*), is the Anna D. Wolf Chair and a professor in the Johns Hopkins University (JHU) School of Nursing, with a joint appointment in the Bloomberg School of Public Health. She is also an inaugural Gilman Scholar at JHU. She is national program director of the Robert Wood Johnson Foundation Nurse Faculty Scholars program. Dr. Campbell has been conducting advocacy policy work and research in the area of violence against women since 1980, with 12 major federally funded research grants and more than 220 articles and 7 books. She is an elected member of the Institute of Medicine (IOM) and the American Academy of Nursing as well as chair of the Board of Directors of Futures without Violence. She served on the Department of Defense Task Force on Domestic Violence and been a consultant to the U.S. Department of Health and Human Services (HHS), Centers for Disease Control and Prevention (CDC), World Health Organization (WHO), and U.S. Agency for International Development. She received the National Friends of the National Institute for Nursing Research (NINR) Research Pathfinder Award, the Sigma Theta Tau International Nurse Researcher Award, and the American Society of Criminology Vollmer Award for advancing justice. Dr. Campbell co-chaired the Steering Committee for the WHO Multicountry Study on Violence Against Women and Women's Health, has been appointed to three IOM/National Academy of Sciences committees evaluating evidence in various aspects of violence against women, and currently serves on the IOM Board on Global Health. In addition, she co-chairs the IOM Forum on Global Violence Prevention. She is also a member of the Fulbright Specialist Roster and does work in collaboration with shelters, governments, criminal justice agencies, schools of nursing, and health care settings in countries such as South Africa, Spain, New Zealand, Australia, Haiti, and the Democratic Republic of the Congo.

E-Shien (Iggy) Chang, M.A., is the research project manager with the Chinese Health, Policy, and Aging Program at Rush Institute for Healthy Aging, Rush University, where she is responsible for managing and coordinating community-engaged, participatory research projects pertaining to the health and well-being of older Chinese adults. In this role, Ms. Chang works as a liaison facilitating research collaborations between Rush and Chinese communities in the greater Chicago area. Prior to joining the team, she worked with various community organizations and advocacy groups in Chicago. Ms. Chang received her M.A. in social sciences from the University of Chicago, and her bachelor's degree in journalism from National Chengchi University, Taiwan.

Marie-Therese Connolly, J.D., is a senior scholar at the Woodrow Wilson International Center for Scholars and a 2011 MacArthur Foundation fellow. She's currently completing a book about elder abuse (W.W. Norton), consulting on a Department of Justice (DOJ)/HHS project to create a roadmap for the elder justice field, and involved in an array of projects designed to advance elder justice. Ms. Connolly has played critical roles in advancing law, policy, research, and public awareness relating to elder abuse. She conceived of and was the original architect of the Elder Justice Act, the only federal law to comprehensively address elder abuse, neglect, and exploitation (enacted in 2010 with the Affordable Care Act). As the founding head of DOJ's Elder Justice and Nursing Home Initiative, she guided theory and strategy in cases against providers that abuse and neglect; launched the first (and still only) ongoing elder justice research grant program through DOJ's National Institute of Justice; launched the federal interagency Elder Justice Working Group; organized the first forum on the medical forensics of elder abuse and numerous other events; and wrote speeches for high-level government officials on elder justice issues, including for members of the Cabinet and Congress. She has testified before Congress and the Elder Justice Coordinating Council (at its inaugural meeting in 2012), is a frequent public speaker and commentator in the media on elder justice issues, and has published articles on elder justice issues in a variety of academic, policy, and news venues publications. Ms. Connolly is a graduate of Stanford University and Northeastern University Law School.

XinQi Dong, M.D., M.P.H. (*Forum Member*), is the director of the Chinese Health, Aging and Policy Program, the associate director of the Rush Institute for Healthy Aging, and an associate professor of medicine, nursing, and behavioral sciences at Rush University Medical Center. Dr. Dong has had longstanding interests in human rights and social justice issues in vulnerable populations, and his research focuses on the epidemiological studies of elder abuse, neglect, and exploitation both in the United States and China, with particular emphasis on adverse health outcomes. Dr. Dong has published extensively on this topic and is currently leading an epidemiological study of 3,000 Chinese older adults to quantify longitudinal relationship among culture factors, elder abuse, and trajectories of psychosocial well-being. Dr. Dong serves on the Editorial Board for *Journal of Elder Abuse and Neglect, Journal of Gerontology Medical Sciences, Gerontology, BioMed Research International, Journal of Aging and Health,* and *Journal of the American Geriatric Society.* As an American Political Science Association (APSA) Congressional Policy Fellow/Health and Aging Policy Fellow, he served as a senior policy and research advisor for the Administration on Aging (AoA)/Administration for Community Living (ACL) and a senior policy advisor for the Centers for Medicare & Medicaid Services (CMS). Dr. Dong is also a recipient of the Paul Beeson Award in Aging, National Physician Advocacy Merit Award, the Nobuo Maeda International Aging and Public Health Research Award, and the Maxwell Pollack Award in Productive Aging. Dr. Dong was elected to be a commissioner for the Commission on Law and Aging of the American Bar Association (ABA), and the Board of Directors for the Chinese American Service League, the largest social services organization in the Midwest serving the needs of Chinese populations. He is a Fellow of the Institute of Medicine of Chicago and a member of the IOM Forum on Global Violence Prevention. He received his B.A. in biology and economics from the University of Chicago, his M.D. in the problem-based curriculum at Rush University College of Medicine, and his M.P.H. in epidemiology at University of Illinois at Chicago. He completed his internal medicine residency and geriatric fellowship at Yale University Medical Center.

Carmel Bitondo Dyer, M.D., is a graduate of Baylor College of Medicine, where she completed her Internal Medicine residency and Geriatrics Fellowship. She founded the geriatrics program at the Harris County Hospital District and the Texas Elder Abuse and Mistreatment Institute. Her research and publications have been in elder mistreatment. She was a delegate to the 2005 White House Conference on Aging and has twice provided testimony to the U.S. Senate on behalf of vulnerable elders. She has received national and local recognition for her teaching abilities, research inroads, and dedication to the health care of older persons. Dr. Dyer joined the University of Texas (UT) Health faculty in 2007 and is professor of medicine and director of the Geriatric and Palliative Medicine Division. She is the interim chief of staff for LBJ Hospital and associate dean of Harris County Programs for UT Health. Dr. Dyer holds the Roy M. and Phyllis Gough Huffington

Chair in Gerontology and is executive director of the UT Health Consortium on Aging.

Terry Fulmer, Ph.D., R.N., F.A.A.N., is professor and dean of the Bouve College of Health Sciences and professor of Public Policy and Urban Affairs in the College of Social Sciences and Humanities at Northeastern University. She received her Bachelor's degree from Skidmore College, her Master's and Doctoral degrees from Boston College, and her Geriatric Nurse Practitioner Post-Master's Certificate from New York University (NYU). She is an elected member of the IOM and currently serves as vice chair of the New York Academy of Medicine. She is an attending nurse and senior nurse in the Munn Center for Nursing Research at Massachusetts General Hospital. Dr. Fulmer is nationally and internationally recognized as a leading expert in geriatrics and is best known for her research on the topic of elder abuse and neglect, which has been funded by the NIA and NINR. She most recently served as the Erline Perkins McGriff Professor of Nursing and founding dean of the New York University College of Nursing. She has held faculty appointments at Boston College, Columbia University, Yale University, and the Harvard Division on Aging. She has served as a visiting professor of nursing at the University of Pennsylvania and Case Western Reserve University. Dr. Fulmer is dedicated to the advancement of intraprofessional health science education and progress in interdisciplinary practice and research. Her clinical appointments have included the Beth Israel Hospital in Boston, the Massachusetts General Hospital, and the NYU-Langone Medical Center. She is a Fellow in the American Academy of Nursing, Gerontological Society of America, and New York Academy of Medicine. She completed a Brookdale National Fellowship and is a Distinguished Practitioner of the National Academies of Practice.

Kathy Greenlee, J.D. (*Forum Member*), serves in the dual roles of administrator of the Administration for Community Living and Assistant Secretary for the Administration on Aging. President Obama appointed her to the latter position as Assistant Secretary for Aging at HHS and she was confirmed by the Senate in 2009. ACL is a new federal agency operating within HHS. ACL brings together into a single entity the AoA, the Office on Disability, and the Administration on Developmental Disabilities. ACL is charged with working with states, tribes, community providers, universities, nonprofit organizations, businesses, and families to help seniors and people with disabilities live in their homes and fully participate in their communities. Assistant Secretary Greenlee believes that people with functional support needs should have the opportunity to live independently in a home of their choosing, receiving appropriate services and supports. She is committed to building the capacity of the national aging and disability networks to better serve older persons, caregivers, and individuals with disabilities. Ms. Greenlee served as Secretary of Aging in Kansas, and before that as the Kansas state long-term care ombudsman. She also served as general counsel of the Kansas Insurance Department and as chief of staff and chief of operations for then-Governor Kathleen Sebelius. Ms. Greenlee is a graduate of the University of Kansas with degrees in business administration and law.

Jeffrey E. Hall, Ph.D., M.S.P.H., M.A., is a behavioral scientist at the CDC Division of Violence Prevention (DVP) of the National Center for Injury Prevention and Control. A medical sociologist by training, he also holds degrees in Epidemiology, General Sociology, and Psychology. His research at the CDC focuses on topics spanning the life course, including infant homicide, youth violence, and elder abuse. He serves as the acting team leader for the Morbidity and Behavioral Surveillance Team in DVP's Surveillance Branch, Principal Investigator for the CDC School Associated Violent Deaths Study, and co-chair of the DVP Youth Violence Workgroup. He is also chair of the CDC Aging and Health Work Group and is a co-lead of the DVP Elder Abuse Workgroup.

Lori L. Jervis, Ph.D., is an associate professor at the University of Oklahoma Department of Anthropology and a director at the Center for Applied Social Research. A cultural/medical anthropologist as well as gerontologist, her work focuses on the intersection of culture, aging, and health. Dr. Jervis has conducted federally funded research on Native American mental and cognitive health, trauma, and violence. She was principal investigator of a collaborative research project funded by the NIA on elder mistreatment among Native Americans in rural reservations and urban contexts. Dr. Jervis's research interests include long-term care, with a focus on nursing homes, as well as rural primary care. She has more than two decades of research experience in gerontological anthropology and 16 years devoted specifically to Native Americans. Dr. Jervis is past president of the Association of Anthropology and Gerontology and a current Advisory Board member for the National Indigenous Elder Justice Initiative. Prior to taking a position at the University of Oklahoma, she was on the faculty at the American Indian and Alaska Native Programs in the Department of Psychiatry at the University of Colorado, Denver. There she served as a principal ethnographer on a major psychiatric epidemiology study, where issues of trauma related to contemporary reservation life and the larger dynamics of cultural trauma emerged as central issues in intergenerational family life. She has published numerous articles in psychiatric anthropology, gerontology, and neuropsychiatry and, with colleagues, developed a measure to improve the assessment of the mistreatment of older Native Americans.

Carole Johnson, M.A., serves on the White House Domestic Policy Council health team working on public health and health care initiatives. She previously served as policy director for the Bureau of Health Professions at the Health Resources and Services Administration in HHS. Prior to joining HHS, she was a lead research scientist and lecturer at the George Washington University's Center for Health Policy Research. Ms. Johnson previously was a senior policy consultant with Health Policy R&D, a policy research and analysis group. She also served as health staff to Sen. Maria Cantwell (D-WA) and Rep. Karen Thurman (D-FL) and on the legislative staff of Rep. Bill Hughes (D-NJ). In addition, she was policy director for the Alliance of Community Health Plans, an association of nonprofit health plans; program officer with the Pew Charitable Trusts Health and Human Services Program; and senior government relations manager with the American Heart Association. She holds a master's degree in government from the University of Virginia.

Alexandre Kalache, Ph.D., M.D., was director of the WHO Department of Ageing and Life Course from 1995 until 2008. Since then, he has been acting as senior policy advisor to the President on Global Ageing at the New York Academy of Medicine and, concomitantly, as a consultant to the municipal and state governments in Rio de Janeiro and the federal government in Brasilia. Under his leadership, WHO launched the Global Movement on Age-Friendly Cities in 2007. He also serves as HelpAge International Global Ambassador on Ageing. This combination of duties indicates the establishment and enhancement of international links, codirecting specific projects based on age-friendly approaches, fostering public–private initiatives on aging, and highlighting the importance of intersectoral action for the full implementation of the Madrid International Plan of Action on Ageing. Over recent years, Dr. Kalache has been in the forefront of the process of strengthening human rights of older people at the international level, most importantly toward the adoption of a United Nations (UN) Convention of Rights of Older People. Previously, Dr. Kalache served as founder and head of the Epidemiology of Ageing Unit at the London School of Hygiene and Tropical Medicine, where he also set up the first European Master's Degree Course on Health Promotion. From 1978 to 1984, Dr. Kalache was a clinical lecturer at the Department of Community Health, Oxford University. He holds several honorary positions from various universities around the world and is a Board member of several professional international associations in gerontology, public health, and geriatric medicine. Dr. Kalache obtained his master's degree in social medicine from the University of London, his M.D. from the Federal University of Rio de Janeiro, and his Ph.D. in epidemiology from the University of Oxford.

Jason Karlawish, M.D., is a professor of medicine, medical ethics, and health policy at the University of Pennsylvania Perelman School of Medicine. He is board certified in geriatric medicine. Dr. Karlawish is a Senior Fellow of the Leonard Davis Institute of Health Economics, a Fellow of the University of Pennsylvania's Institute on Aging, director of the Penn Neurodegenerative Disease Ethics and Policy Program, and associate director of the Penn Memory Center. He is also director of the Alzheimer's Disease Center's Education, Recruitment, and Retention Core. His research focuses on neuroethics and policy. He has investigated issues in dementia drug development, informed consent, quality of life, research and treatment decision making, and voting by persons with dementia.

Mark Lachs, M.D., M.P.H., is director of geriatrics for the New York Presbyterian Health System, co-chief of the Division of Geriatric Medicine and Gerontology at the Weill Medical College of Cornell University, and a tenured clinical professor of medicine at the College. A graduate of the University of Pennsylvania and the NYU School of Medicine, he completed a residency in internal medicine at The Hospital of the University of Pennsylvania and is board certified in internal medicine. In 1988, he became a Robert Wood Johnson Clinical Scholar at Yale, where he also earned an M.P.H. in chronic disease epidemiology and added qualification in geriatric medicine from the American Board of Internal Medicine. He spent 4 years on the Yale faculty before coming to Cornell to lead the Geriatrics Program. Dr. Lachs' major area of interest is the disenfranchised elderly, and he has published widely in the areas of elder abuse and neglect, Adult Protective Services, the measurement of functional status, ethics, and the financing of health care. His many honors and awards include an American College of Physicians Teaching and Research Scholarship, an NIA Academic Leadership Award, and a Paul Beeson Physician Faculty Scholarship (the country's preeminent career development award in aging) from the American Federation for Aging Research through funding from the John A. Hartford Foundation and the Alliance for Aging Research. He is also the recipient of RO1 funding from the NIH to study the impact of crime on the physical and emotional health of older adults. He was asked to serve as an advisor for WHO on elder abuse. Recently, he has been instrumental in advocating for the creation of a dedicated elder abuse center in New York City. In 2010, Penguin Viking published his book *Treat Me, Not My Age: A Doctor's Guide to Getting the Best Care as You or a Loved One Gets Older* (www.treatmenotmyage.com).

Gill Livingston, MBChB, FRCPsych, M.D., is a professor in psychiatry of older people in the Mental Health Science Unit in University College of London and consultant old age psychiatrist. She is interested in clinical research in dementia—from epidemiology to pragmatic randomized controlled trials; from diagnosis to end of life. Current funded research includes the START study (STrAtegies for RelaTives) of coping studies for family careers; a systematic review of effectiveness and cost-effectiveness of non-drug interventions for agitation in people with dementia; and improving end-of-life care for dementia in care homes. She has been working in research in elder abuse for many years and most of this has been with her colleague Claudia Cooper.

Ronald Long, J.D., is the senior vice president and director of Regulatory Affairs at Wells Fargo Advisors, LLC. In this role, Mr. Long works with key business and support units to foster substantial engagement in and awareness of the changing regulatory and legislative environment. He leads the firm's efforts to comment on rule changes and helps shape laws impacting the securities industry. Mr. Long joined Wells Fargo Advisors through the merger of Wachovia and Wells Fargo. He joined Wachovia in 2002 and worked in the legal department, leading the team focused on regulatory inquiries. Prior to joining the firm, Mr. Long was district administrator of the Securities and Exchange Commission's Philadelphia District Office from 1997 to 2002. He joined the Commission staff in 1990 as an attorney in the Division of Enforcement. Mr. Long later assumed the position of counselor to Chair Arthur Levitt. Mr. Long attended Williams College and received his J.D. from Georgetown University Law Center.

Susan Lynch, J.D., M.P.H., LL.M., is a trial attorney at DOJ, where she leads national investigations and civilly prosecutes long-term care facilities for failing to adequately care for their residents. Ms. Lynch sits on the Federal Elder Justice Interagency Working Group, which addresses policy issues such as elder abuse and financial exploitation. Ms. Lynch serves as an adjunct professor of law at the George Washington University Law School, where she has taught since the fall of 2000. Prior to joining DOJ, Ms. Lynch was a litigation associate in private practice in Washington, DC. Ms. Lynch received her B.A. from Dartmouth College, her J.D. from the Indiana University Maurer School of Law, where she served as editor-in-chief of the *Indiana Journal of Global Legal Studies*, and her LL.M. (master's of law in advocacy) with Distinction from the Georgetown University Law Center. Ms. Lynch received her M.P.H. from the Johns Hopkins Bloomberg School of Public Health, where she was inducted into the Delta Omega Public Health Honor Society.

Brigid McCaw, M.D., M.S., M.P.H., FACP (*Forum Member*), is medical director for the Family Violence Prevention Program at Kaiser Permanente (KP). Her teaching, research, and publications focus on developing a health systems response to intimate partner violence and the impact of such violence on health status and mental health. She is a Fellow of the American College of Physicians. KP, a large, nonprofit integrated health care organization serving 8.6 million members in nine states and the District of Columbia, has implemented one of the most comprehensive health care responses to domestic violence in the United States. The nationally recognized "systems-model" approach is available across the continuum of care, including outpatient, emergency, and inpatient care; advice and call centers; and chronic care programs. The electronic medical record includes clinician tools to facilitate recognition, referrals, resources, and follow-up for patients experiencing domestic violence and provides data for quality improvement measures. Over the past decade, identification of domestic violence has increased five-fold, with most members identified in the ambulatory rather than the acute care setting. The majority of identified patients receive follow-up mental health services. KP also provides prevention, outreach, and domestic violence resources for its workforce. Violence prevention is an important focus for KP community benefit investments and research studies. The KP program, under the leadership of Dr. McCaw, has received several national awards.

Tara McMullen, M.P.H., Ph.D.(c), is a health analyst at CMS in the Quality Measurement & Health Assessment Group. Ms. McMullen is the health analyst for Nursing Homes and Home Health, working on quality measurement development for the Nursing Home and Home Health Compare sites. Ms. McMullen is a core team member of the CMS initiative, the National Partnership to Improve Dementia Care, the agency-wide initiative of the Adverse Drug Events Task Force, and the CMS Elder Maltreatment Initiative. Moreover, Ms. McMullen is a technical expert for the Pharmacy Quality Alliance's Technical Expert Panel on pharmacy-related measurement development. Ms. McMullen has published in the *New England Journal of Medicine*, the *Journal for Geriatrics and Gerontology Education*, the *Journal of Nursing Measurement*, and the *International Journal of Aging in Society*.

Charles P. Mouton, M.D., M.S., is senior vice president for health affairs and dean of the School of Medicine at Meharry Medical College in Nashville, Tennessee. He is also professor of family and community medicine at Meharry Medical College and professor of medical education and administration at Vanderbilt University School of Medicine. As dean, Dr. Mouton serves as chief academic and administrative officer of the school and is responsible for academic programs, student affairs, graduate medical education, curriculum development and management, and financial management of Meharry's largest academic unit. As senior vice president of health affairs, he is responsible for overseeing, enhancing, and expanding Meharry clinical programs, working closely with key stakeholders of the College and within the community. Dr. Mouton is board certified in family medicine and holds a certificate of added qualifications in geriatrics. Additionally, he is a certified medical director. He received his bachelor's degree in engineering from Howard University. He also holds an M.S. in epidemiology and an M.S. in clinical epidemiology from the Harvard University School of Public Health. He received his M.D. from the Howard University College of Medicine, completed a Family Practice Residency at Prince George's Hospital Center in Cheverly, Maryland, and finished a Geriatrics Fellowship at The George Washington Medical Center. Dr. Mouton's major areas of research interests are elderly mistreatment violence in older women, health promotion and disease prevention in minority elders (especially exercise for the elderly), ethnicity and aging, and quality health care for minorities.

James G. O'Brien, M.D., is professor and the Margaret Dorward Smock Endowed Chair in Geriatrics, as well as chair of the Department of Family and Geriatric Medicine at the University of Louisville in Kentucky. He did his undergraduate and medical training at University College in Dublin, Ireland, Family Medicine Residency at Saginaw Cooperative Hospital, and Fellowship in Geriatrics at Duke University. He is an AoA member and Fellow of the Gerontological Society of America and the American Geriatrics Society, received the "Champion for the Aging Award" by Elderserve, Inc., of Louisville, Kentucky, and is an inductee into the Arnold P. Gold Honors Society for Humanism in Medicine. Since 2003, he has served on the Governor's Task Force on Abuse & Neglect of Elderly for the Commonwealth of Kentucky. Dr. O'Brien was editor of a 1999 issue of the *Journal of Elder Abuse & Neglect* titled Self-Neglect: Challenges for Helping Professionals and was primary author or co-author of three of the articles. He has more than 50 publications in peer-reviewed journals, 2 textbooks, and 15 chapters, and serves on the Editorial Board of *Journal of Elder Abuse and Neglect*. He was inducted as a fellow in The Royal College of Physicians of Ireland in March 2011.

Elizabeth Podnieks, Ed.D., M.S., is a professor emeritus at Ryerson University. She conducted the *National Survey of Abuse of the Elderly in Canada* in 1991. This landmark survey was the first to be national in scope and marked an important step for understanding the extent of the problem of elder abuse. A pioneer in raising awareness of elder abuse within faith communities and among children and youth, Dr. Podnieks has conducted research and published in these areas. She represented Canada in the WHO/International Network for the Prevention of Elder Abuse (INPEA) Global

Response to Elder Abuse and Missing Voices. She has published and presented papers at the national and international levels. She is on the Editorial Board of the *Journal of Elder Abuse and Neglect*, and has served on the Editorial Board of the *Journal of Gerontological Nursing*. Dr. Podnieks is founder of the Canadian Network for the Prevention of Elder Abuse and is a founding member and immediate past president of the INPEA. She is an Honorary Board Member of the National Committee for the Prevention of Elder Abuse. Dr. Podnieks is currently working with Dr. Pamela Teaster and Dr. Georgia Anetzberger on the second phase of the global study, The Worldwide Face of Elder Abuse. Other research activities include working with the Registered Nurses Association of Ontario on developing Best Practice Guidelines on Elder Abuse Awareness, Prevention and Intervention. Dr. Podnieks was the founder of World Elder Abuse and Awareness Day (WEAAD) in 2003. In 2012 she developed World Day in Cyberspace. She was awarded the Order of Canada and the Queen Elizabeth II Diamond Jubilee Medal in recognition for work in the field of elder abuse. Her degrees include a bachelor of nursing, master's in environmental science, and an Ed.D. in sociology.

Kathleen Quinn is the executive director of the National Adult Protective Services Association (NAPSA), the only national organization representing Adult Protective Services (APS) programs, professionals, and clients. NAPSA, which has more than 600 members, is funded by AoA for the first National APS Resource Center. NAPSA also provides the only annual national conference on elder abuse, abuse of younger adults with disabilities, and APS. Ms. Quinn previously served as policy advisor on senior issues to the Illinois Attorney General, and as the chief of the Bureau of Elder Rights for the Illinois Department on Aging, where she administered the statewide Elder Abuse and Neglect Program and the Long Term Care Ombudsman Program. Earlier she worked with the Illinois Coalition Against Domestic Violence, where she was responsible for the first statewide training of law enforcement and prosecutors on domestic violence and the then–newly enacted Illinois Domestic Violence Act.

Daniel Reingold, M.S.W., J.D., is president and chief executive officer of The Hebrew Home at Riverdale in New York City. The Hebrew Home is a nonsectarian, not-for-profit geriatric service organization that provides residential health care, senior housing communities, and a full spectrum of home care, rehabilitation, and adult day and overnight respite programs offered by its ElderServe community services division. The Hebrew Home serves more than 7,000 older people in the Bronx, Manhattan, and Westchester County. In 2005, it established The Harry and Jeanette Weinberg Center for Elder Abuse Prevention, the nation's first comprehensive elder abuse shelter.

Prior to joining The Hebrew Home in 1990, Mr. Reingold was an attorney in private practice representing nonprofit organizations. Mr. Reingold serves on the Boards of Directors of the Continuing Care Leadership Coalition, the Greater New York Hospital Association, and the Association of Jewish Aging Services. Mr. Reingold received a B.A. from Hobart College, an M.S.W. from Columbia University, and a law degree from the Benjamin N. Cardozo School of Law of Yeshiva University.

Charles Sabatino, J.D., is the director of the ABA's Commission on Law and Aging in Washington, DC, where since 1984 he has been responsible for the ABA Commission's research, project development, consultation, and education in the areas of health law, long-term care, guardianship and capacity issues, surrogate decision making, legal services delivery for the elderly, and professional ethics. Mr. Sabatino has written and spoken extensively on capacity issues, surrogate decision making, and health care policy. Mr. Sabatino is also a part-time adjunct professor at Georgetown University Law Center, where he has taught about law and aging since 1987. He is a Fellow and former president of the National Academy of Elder Law Attorneys. He received his A.B. from Cornell University and his J.D. from Georgetown University Law Center and is a member of the Virginia and Washington, DC, bars.

Judith A. Salerno, M.D., M.S., is the former Leonard D. Schaeffer Executive Officer of the IOM of the National Academies. Dr. Salerno was the executive director and chief operating officer of the Institute. She was responsible for managing the IOM's research and policy programs and guiding the Institute's operations on a daily basis. Prior to coming to the IOM, Dr. Salerno was Deputy Director of NIA at NIH, HHS. She oversaw more than $1 billion in aging research conducted and supported annually by NIA, including research on Alzheimer's and other neurodegenerative diseases, frailty and function in late life, and the social, behavioral and demographic aspects of aging. As NIA's senior geriatrician, Dr. Salerno was vitally interested in improving the health and well-being of older persons, and designed public–private initiatives to address aging stereotypes, novel approaches to support training of new investigators in aging, and award-winning programs to communicate health and research advances to the public. Before joining NIA in 2001, Dr. Salerno directed the continuum of Geriatrics and Extended Care programs across the nation for the U.S. Department of Veterans Affairs (VA), Washington, DC. While at VA, she launched widely recognized national initiatives for pain management and improving end-of-life care. Prior to this appointment, Dr. Salerno was Associate Chief of Staff at the VA Medical Center in Washington, DC, where she developed and implemented innovative approaches to geriatric primary care and coordinated area-wide geriatric medicine training. Dr. Salerno also co-founded the Washington, DC, Area Geriatric Education Center Consortium, a collaboration of more than 160 educational and community organizations within the Baltimore-Washington region. The consortium generates educational opportunities for professionals serving the aging. Earlier in her career, Dr. Salerno was a Senior Clinical Investigator at NIA, implementing clinical research protocols for patients with Alzheimer's disease and hypertension. Dr. Salerno also served on numerous boards and national committees concerned with health care issues ranging from the quality of care in long-term care to the future of the geriatric workforce and currently serves of the boards of several arts organizations. Dr. Salerno earned her M.D. degree from Harvard Medical School in 1985 and a master of science degree in health policy from the Harvard School of Public Health in 1976. She also holds a certificate of added qualifications in geriatric medicine and was associate clinical professor of health care sciences and of medicine at the George Washington University until 2001.

Kimberly Schwartz is a nurse consultant and the program manager for the CMS Physician Quality Reporting System (PQRS) clinical quality measures, eRx lead and coordinates the alignment of the measures with the other quality reporting programs within CMS. Ms. Schwartz has more than 20 years' experience in the areas of neonatal and trauma nursing. She has extensive knowledge of clinical quality measures using different data sources and reporting mechanisms. Ms. Schwartz is a registered nurse. She has a B.S.N. from Towson University and is working on her master's in nursing.

Gregory R. Shaw has a science and health administration background and, until assuming the position of director, International and Corporate Relations of the International Federation on Ageing (IFA) in 2003, held senior management positions within the Australian Commonwealth Department Health and Ageing. Prior to joining the IFA, he managed residential and community aging programs in Western Australia. His long career with the Australian government included management of the Compliance, Complaint and Accountability Section of the Department and responsibility for the regulatory arena associated with quality of care and certification programs in both residential and community care services. His earlier work focused on policy development and program implementation supporting the aged-care needs of rural and remote communities throughout Northern Australia. An advocate of the aging needs of marginalized community groups, he worked with many Aboriginal and ethnic communities, resulting in the establishment of aged-care homes and community services. Since joining the IFA, Mr. Shaw has had responsibility for development of the Building Capacity in Health Care Programs in Africa and worked closely with the South African Human Rights Commission to establish an older person's forum. In 2010 he worked with the government of Mauritius on the establishment of an Observatory on Ageing. He represents the IFA at the United Nations, works closely with government, and has responsibility for IFA elder abuse initiatives. These initiatives have included the development of educational toolkits targeted to youth; in 2011 he convened an International Forum on Sexual Safety of Older Women, and in 2013 led a high-level meeting to examine issues of financial abuse of Canadian seniors. In 2013, he worked with other civil society organizations on the global thematic consultations on population dynamics, post-2015 development agenda to ensure the needs of older people are recognized.

Paul Smocer is president of The Financial Services Roundtable, and oversees BITS, the technology policy division. Previously, he served as president of Financial Services Technology Consortium (FSTC) and worked to integrate BITS's and FSTC's work. Mr. Smocer joined the Roundtable in 2008 as vice president of security, leading BITS's work in promoting the safety and soundness of financial institutions through best practices and successful strategies for developing secure infrastructures, products, and services. Prior to BITS, Mr. Smocer focused on technology risk management at Bank of New York Mellon (BNY Mellon) and led information security at the former Mellon Financial Corporation. He was previously the chief information security officer and manager of Mellon Financial Corporation's Technology Assurance Services Division, responsible for information security and technology risk management. Mr. Smocer began his career at Mellon when he joined its Information Technology Audit group, for which he worked until he left to join another Pittsburgh-based institution. Mr. Smocer started up that institution's information technology audit function until he became chief auditor. He was ultimately responsible for the internal audit, risk management, and corporate compliance functions. He returned to Mellon as a division manager in its Audit and Risk Review Department, where he managed the technology audit group. While at BNY Mellon and at Mellon, he was actively engaged with BITS as a member of its Vendor Management Working Group, chair of the Security Steering Committee, and chair of the former Operational Risk Committee. Mr. Smocer has more than 30 years of experience in technology, security, and control functions. He is a magna cum laude graduate of Indiana University of Pennsylvania with a degree in business management, concentrating in business systems.

Joy Solomon, J.D., is director and managing attorney of The Harry and Jeanette Weinberg Center for Elder Abuse Prevention, the nation's first emergency shelter for elder abuse victims. Ms. Solomon cofounded the Weinberg Center in 2004. She was previously director of Elder Abuse

Services at the Pace Women's Justice Center, a nonprofit legal advocacy and training center based at Pace University Law School. Prior to joining the Women's Justice Center, she investigated and prosecuted a variety of crimes, including child abuse, fraud, and elder abuse, as an assistant district attorney in Manhattan, where she served for 8 years. She is a Board member of National Committee for the Prevention of Elder Abuse (NCPEA); on the Executive Committee of the Elder Law Section of the New York State Bar Association, where she is chair of the Elder Abuse Committee; and on the Advisory Board of the New York City Elder Abuse Center, of which she was a founder. In 2010, she received The New York State Bar Association award for Excellence in Public Service.

Susan B. Somers, J.D., practices in areas including civil rights, family, and elder issues. She holds a Certificate of Gerontology Studies. She served as assistant deputy attorney general for the state of New York, heading a section of Consumer Frauds and the Elder Protection Unit. She was state director of the Office of Children and Family Services (OCFS) Bureau of Adults Services from 2002 until 2007. She has served as Secretary General of the International Network for the Prevention of Elder Abuse since 2003. Her focus in human rights is to end abuse, neglect, and violence against vulnerable older persons globally, addressing harmful cultural and traditional practices. Ms. Somers chairs the Elder Abuse Subcommittee of the NGO Committee on Ageing, New York. She participated in the first United Nations Department of Public Information (UN DPI) Briefing on Social Isolation. As part of a National Caregiver training cosponsored by the Nepal Ministry of Women, Children and Social Welfare, and the National Network of Senior Citizens Organization of Nepal, she presented on elder abuse prevention, caretaker stress, and dealing with difficult behaviors of persons with Alzheimer's and other types of dementia. Ms. Somers earned a J.D. from Albany Law School.

Sidney M. Stahl, Ph.D., served as the chief of the Individual Behavioral Processes Branch in the Division of Behavioral and Social Research at NIA from 1996 until his retirement in 2012. As branch chief, Dr. Stahl was responsible for the group that set NIA's research agendas on health and behavior, cognitive functioning, emotional well-being, and integrative approaches to the study of social and psychological factors as they impact older persons. The Branch focused primarily on maintaining health and well-being over the lifecourse. During his tenure at NIA, Dr. Stahl played a leading role in promoting diversity in aging research, most notably through his stewardship of the Resource Centers on Minority Aging Research. He was directly responsible for building NIA's research programs on elder mistreatment, long-term care, caregiving, and behavioral medicine. The

Gerontological Society of America (GSA) chose Dr. Stahl as the 2012 recipient of the Donald P. Kent Award. This distinguished honor is given annually to a GSA member who best exemplifies the highest standards for professional leadership in gerontology through teaching, service, and interpretation of gerontology to the larger society. Prior to his career at NIH, Dr. Stahl served as a researcher and professor of medical sociology and social gerontology at Purdue University for more than 20 years. He published extensively on the health of older Americans, social factors in chronic disease, minority aging health, and statistical methods for the measurement of health in aging populations. He served as consultant to WHO in Geneva and Beijing and as a Visiting Scholar at Cambridge University in England. Dr. Stahl is active professionally in GSA, for which he is a Fellow, and the American Sociological Association, for which he was on the Councils of the Section on Aging and the Life Course and the Section on Medical Sociology.

Lori Stiegel, J.D., senior attorney, joined the ABA Commission on Law and Aging staff in 1989. She has developed and directed all of the Commission's work on elder abuse, including numerous federal grant projects for DOJ and HHS, focusing on legal interventions or laws governing non-legal interventions. She is the author or co-author of numerous books, manuals, curriculums, and articles, including *Power of Attorney Abuse: What States Can Do About It—A Comparison of Current State Laws with the New Uniform Power of Attorney Act* (2008); *Elder Abuse Detection and Intervention: A Collaborative Approach* (Springer, 2007); *Undue Influence: The Criminal Justice Response* (YWCA of Omaha, 2006); and *Recommended Guidelines for State Courts Handling Cases Involving Elder Abuse* (ABA, 1995). Ms. Stiegel was a member of the National Academy of Sciences' Study Panel on the Risk and Prevalence of Elder Abuse and contributed to the panel's groundbreaking report *Elder Mistreatment: Abuse, Neglect, and Exploitation in an Aging America* (NRC, 2003).

Pamela B. Teaster, M.A., Ph.D., is a professor in the Department of Health Behavior and director of Doctoral Studies in the College of Public Health at the University of Kentucky. She directs the Kentucky Justice Center for Elders and Vulnerable Adults and is president of the Kentucky Guardianship Association. She serves on the Editorial Boards of the *Journal of Applied Gerontology* and the *Journal of Elder Abuse and Neglect*. Dr. Teaster is a Fellow of the Gerontological Society of America and the Association for Gerontology in Higher Education, a recipient of the Rosalie Wolf Award for Research on Elder Abuse, the Outstanding Affiliate Member Award (Kentucky Guardianship Association), and the Distinguished Educator Award (Kentucky Association for Gerontology). She is the author of more than 100 peer-reviewed articles, reports, books, and book chapters.

Agnes Tiwari, Ph.D., R.N., is professor and head of the School of Nursing at the Li Ka Shing Faculty of Medicine of the University of Hong Kong (UHK). She is a nurse with extensive experience in clinical practice, administration, education, and research. Prevention of family violence is the focus of her practice, research, teaching, and advocacy work. Recognizing the need for primary prevention of violence in the community, she has collaborated with professionals in primary care and community settings to provide education and support to parents, expectant couples, and elder caregivers for the promotion of harmonious family relationships. She has received grants and awards for her research and service projects, and published extensively on violence prevention and intervention. In recognition of her contributions to research and education on violence prevention, she was selected as a fellow of the American Academy of Nursing in 2010, awarded the Women of Influence 2011 by the American Chamber of Commerce in Hong Kong, and received the UHK Research Output Prize in 2011.

Javier Vasquez, LL.M., J.D., has practiced international human rights law with particular emphasis on reproductive rights, the rights of indigenous peoples, disability rights, and the human rights of older persons, among others, for more than 15 years. Currently, he is the human rights law advisor with the Pan American Health Organization (PAHO)/WHO. He advises PAHO Member States, civil society, multilateral organizations, and universities and international/regional treaty bodies (e.g., the Inter-American Commission on Human Rights, or IACHR) on human rights issues and strategies and on the formulation/review of national laws, policies, programs, services, and plans in a manner consistent with international and regional human rights treaties, international case law, and IACHR jurisprudence. He also drafts intergovernmental resolutions and plans and conducts capacity-building consultations and presentations for mainstreaming human rights in PAHO's Secretariat and countries. Mr. Vasquez has conducted official visits to 28 countries and participated in the negotiations/formulations of several international/regional human rights treaties and standards, including the current draft Inter-American Convention on the Rights of Older Persons.

Edwin L. Walker, J.D., is the Deputy Assistant Secretary for Program Operations with AoA. He serves as the chief career official for the federal agency responsible for advocating on behalf of older Americans. He guides and promotes the development of home- and community-based long-term care programs, policies, and services designed to afford older people and their caregivers the ability to age with dignity and independence and to have a broad array of options for an enhanced quality of life. This includes the promotion and implementation of evidence-based prevention interventions proven effective in avoiding or delaying the onset of chronic disease and illness. He has served as the primary liaison with Congress on legislation related to aging services and programs. Prior to joining AoA, Mr. Walker served as director of the Missouri Division of Aging, responsible for administering a comprehensive set of human service programs for older persons and adults with disabilities. He received a B.A. in mass media arts from Hampton University and a J.D. from the University of Missouri–Columbia School of Law.

Robert B. Wallace, M.D., M.Sc., is the Irene Ensminger Stecher professor of epidemiology and internal medicine at the University of Iowa Colleges of Public Health and Medicine, and director of the University's Center on Aging. He has been a member of the U.S. Preventive Services Task Force, and the National Advisory Council on Aging of NIH. He is an elected Member of the IOM, and past chair of the IOM Board on Health Promotion and Disease Prevention and Board on the Health of Select Populations. He recently received the Walsh McDermott award for distinguished service to the IOM. He is the author or co-author of more than 400 publications and 25 book chapters, and has been the editor of 4 books, including the current edition of *Maxcy-Rosenau-Last Public Health and Preventive Medicine*. Dr. Wallace's research interests are in clinical and population epidemiology, and focus on the causes and prevention of disabling conditions among older persons. He has had substantial experience in the conduct of both observational cohort studies of older persons and clinical trials, including preventive interventions related to fracture, cancer, coronary disease, and women's health. For more than 17 years, he was the site principal investigator for the Women's Health Initiative, a set of national intervention trials exploring the prevention of breast and colon cancer and coronary disease. He is a co-investigator of the Health and Retirement Study and the National Health and Aging Trends Study, two national cohort studies of the health, social, and economic status of older Americans.

Mark Yaffe, B.Sc., M.D., C.M., MClSc, CCFP, FCFP, is a tenured full professor in the McGill University Department of Family Medicine in Montreal. As a principal or co–principal investigator, Dr. Yaffe has received research grants totaling more than $3.7 million. Research topics have included anticipatory guidance models for the middle-age portion of the lifespan; doctor–patient relationships; interdisciplinary health care; anxiety and depression management; delivery of primary health care; family caregiving; and elder abuse. He served as principal investigator on an interdisciplinary team that developed and validated the Elder Abuse Suspicion Index. He is an elected member of the Board of Directors of the Canadian Network for Prevention of Elder Abuse and the director of training for the International

Network for Prevention of Elder Abuse. At McGill University, he teaches at the medical undergraduate, postgraduate, continuing professional education/faculty development levels. He also conducts master's and Ph.D.-level thesis supervision. He has also served as family medicine postgraduate residency program director. His accomplishments in education have been recognized by early induction into the McGill University Faculty of Medicine Honor List for Educational Excellence. In 2007 he was the Inaugural Recipient of the Prize of Excellence for the Advancement of Family Medicine Education of the Quebec College of Family Physicians and the College of Family Physicians of Canada. At St. Mary's Hospital Center, he has been chief of the Department of Family Medicine and director of the teaching Family Medicine Center. Dr. Yaffe is an honorary fellow of the College of Family Physicians of Canada.

Elsie Yan, Ph.D., is an assistant professor in the Department of Social Work and Social Administration, UHK°. Her research interests include domestic violence, mainly focusing on factors and impacts associated with elder abuse and intimate partner violence in older couples. She is also conducting research on dementia care and elder sexuality. Her publications appeared in *International Psychogeriatrics*, *International Journal of Geriatric Psychiatry*, *Journal of Family Violence*, and *Journal of Interpersonal Violence*, and others.